# THINK
# SLIM

## THE SEVEN-STEP PROGRAMME TO SLIM-FITNESS

### EVE BROCK

This book is dedicated to everyone who wants to become slimmer, fitter and enjoy life and scrumptious food too; and to all those Think Slimmers who are already Doing It, and have taught me while I have taught them.

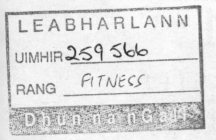

Published in 1992 by Vermilion
an imprint of Ebury Press
Random Century House
20 Vauxhall Bridge Road
London SW1V 2SA

First published 1992

Design: Dennis Barker
Illustrations: Sarah-Jayne Handley

A catalogue record for this book is available from the British
Library.

ISBN: 0 09 175431 3

Typeset in Linotron Sabon by Tek Art Ltd, Croydon, Surrey
Printed and bound in Great Britain by Mackays of Chatham plc, Kent

# CONTENTS

## ACKNOWLEDGEMENTS

To Him Indoors who provided me with low-calorie sustenance (and an occasional lemon meringue pie), and no-calorie loving support while I toiled over this book. Also to Dixie the Dog who took me for inspiring, minus-calorie walks and ate up my high-fat egg yolks.

## *This book is for you if* . . .

- You are overweight and unhappy about it

- You think you can't be Slim

- You want to fit into your too-tight clothes

- You think you'll go on a Diet – tomorrow

- You think you're a Dieting Disaster

- You are thinking of dieting for the first time

- You feel miserable at the very thought of another diet

- You feel enthusiastic about dieting but doubtful you will become slim and stay slim

- Your doctor has advised you to lose weight

- You sometimes think that life is something that 'happens' to you, while you comfort yourself with another biscuit

- You think your slimming may be sabotaged by Real Life Problems, such as a difficult partner; an 'ex' who's still making waves; a crying baby, tantruming toddler or sulky teenager; crotchety customers, a bully-boss, work deadlines; a smothering mother; a critical dad; demanding dependants; a broken washing machine; impossible housing payments; brain-bashing boredom; aching loneliness

- You want to be slimmer and fitter . . .

# IF YOU THINK YOU CAN'T BE SLIM, THINK AGAIN . . .

I used to think I couldn't be slim and stay slim. I used to think – while sweltering in a pink-sprigged shapeless tent that masqueraded as a summer frock – that I was doomed to yo-yo from super-slim size 10 to barrel-shaped out-size.

I used to think that slim people were 'lucky'; that the great people-designer in the sky had played malevolent tricks on me, to slow down my metabolism and denude me of willpower.

I used to think that life would be awful if I had to restrict my eating forever.

I used to think that the solution to losing weight was in the latest miracle diet book, and I devoured diets like Belgian chocolates, but neither diets nor the Belgians succeeded in getting and keeping me slim.

I deprived myself, berated myself, was gripped by guilt and tension, repeatedly went on and off diets – and my weight went down and up. I said no to my favourite foods, no to the cup that cheers; waiting to be thin and dancing to the tune of the diet experts like an unco-ordinated, overweight, programmed puppet. Occasionally, in spasmodic fits of enthusiasm, I exercised my beleaguered body, trying in vain to bash and burn it into thinness. I was thin, sometimes. Often I was overweight and struggling.

I used to think there was no end to this constant battle.

I used to think wrong.

Now I Think Slim. I am permanently slim.

I discovered that the difference between a dieting disaster and a successful slimmer is in the way she/he thinks – about food, about slimming, and about her/his lifestyle. It is our thinking that determines what we eat, how much we eat, and how we live our lives.

This book aims to show you how you can change your thinking to change yourself into a successful slimmer.

If you can Think – you can slim. You can learn to Think Slim, as I and others have done.

Think Slim is not a miracle diet. It means learning how to apply your think-power to drop out of the Diet Trap and start winning at slimming by adopting a slim-fit lifestyle that will last for a lifetime.

To Think Slim, you:
- throw out the diet books, and the guilt and diet-think that goes with them
- think about: your thinking, your eating habits, food and nourishment, your lifestyle, relaxation, exercise
- use a civilised system of eating and drinking which includes your favourite foods in moderation and which nourishes your body
- aim to be slim-fit rather than thin. Being slim-fit means being slim enough and fit enough to really enjoy and make the most of your life
- see slimming as a problem-solving activity. Overcome the obstacles to your slimming by looking for solutions, not excuses.

In order to understand Think Slim, think about this drawing:

What do you see?

You can see either a vase, or two faces in profile.

Just as you can *choose* what to see, you can *choose* what to think:

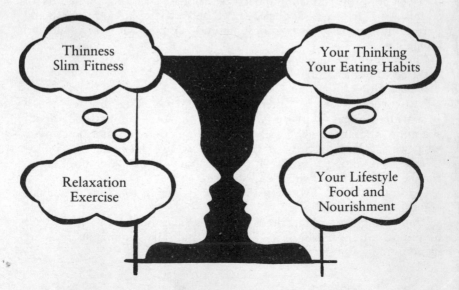

This book is not about how to diet, but how to live; not about how to deprive yourself but how to make the most of your life. Human beings are naturally pleasure-seeking creatures, and this fact of life needs to be incorporated into any slimming regime, or it will fail.

This book sets out the Seven Steps to Slim-fitness, and helps you to help yourself.

First, read my story and the success stories of others who have learned to Think Slim, then learn how to apply your thought power to becoming slim-fit.

## MY STORY

I love clothes, almost as much as I love food. Also, I hate being overweight and I hate being on diets. Finally, I have managed to juggle all those into the best of all worlds by Thinking Slim. Nowadays, I'm slim, don't diet, enjoy my food and save all my pennies to buy clothes. I'll tell you my story.

Perhaps it's not surprising that it was a Posh Frock that started me off, some ten years ago, on that last diet. Another diet. I was an expert dieter. Not that I was slim – well not very often, that is. I was a yo-yo dieter. For fifteen years. My wardrobe was bulging with 'fat' clothes and 'thin' clothes, yet I had hardly anything to wear at any one time.

It was just before Christmas that I spotted the Posh Frock: a strapless, bright burgundy evening dress, and I loved it. I struggled into it in a trice. It clung a little tightly, but I dismissed that depressing thought. I pirouetted and became more confident. Not too tight! When was I going to wear it? We had no formal occasion over Christmas. Practicality won. I handed it back, sadly.

But in January, the Invitation arrived. Dress: Formal. I dashed back for the Posh Frock, with husband in tow. It was still there, waiting for me. On it went, well, almost. None of the zip would fasten. I couldn't have put on that much weight over Christmas! But I knew that I could. The assistant helpfully offered to order me a size 16.

Realism set in. How could I, at only 4 feet 10¾ inches tall, look glamorous in a size 16 strapless dress? A barrel in burgundy!

My husband had an answer. 'We'll take the size 12,' he declared, with an eyebrow raised to me.

I nodded. I'd diet. Again.

I did. Cinderella wore the dress and went to the Ball. And even, later, altered it to a size 10.

But this time there was a different ending – happier ever after. For after losing my excess 2½ stones/16 kilos, I finally dropped out of the Diet Trap, and using the Think Slim strategies, stayed a slim-winner.

First, I took time out to think about my situation. In the past I had been too busy doing and hurrying (and getting fat and dieting) to do much thinking. Now, I thought to myself: 'This fat-thin swing and the yo-yo dieting is absolutely crazy.'

This was a thought revelation to me – and it was based on logical and realistic thinking. I thought on, in the same thought-style (logical and realistic): 'Now that I'm slim I need a system to live by, forever. What can I do?'

I had often read the totally sensible advice to only ever eat when truly hungry and cut out all chocolate, creamy and sweet foods, but I knew that this was no answer for a fallible human like me with my lust for just those fabulous favourite foods. The eternal dilemma: life's too short to live without foodie treats, but it's also too short to live it fat, or on dismally reoccurring diets.

My answer was that instead of 'going back to my normal (fat-making) eating' as I usually did at the triumphant end of a diet, I could simply continue with the eating and exercise patterns that I had recently adopted to get myself slim: that is, choosing wisely those foods that nourished my body, and including my favourite wonderful treats in moderation – and only at the weekends. Even I could survive five stringent eating days each week if I knew that the weekend with its wonderful foodie treats was coming. So, one of my Think Slim philosophies was born: 'If it's Lemon Meringue Pie, it must be Saturday.'

Exercise had helped me to slim, and needed to be built into my routine. 'On yer bike' became my catchphrase and habit; never, never do I ask myself 'Shall I?' for I know that I might answer 'I'll not bother!' So, every morning, before work, I get onto my exercise bike accompanied by an absorbing book or magazine.

My ideas were further developed as I studied for twelve months on a course in Human Relations and counselling. Slimming was never mentioned in my text books or seminars, but so much of what I learned about the psychological connection between human thinking and behaviour applied to slimming. I recognised that to become slim and stay slim we first need to change how we think. I was fascinated by the subject and started sharing the ideas with others in my own slimming groups.

I now explain to those slimmers what I explain here; that a diet is not the answer to their weight problems. It can be replaced with 'slimming', a process of losing weight in a wiser, more civilised and more enjoyable way. Yes, it's probably slower for weight-loss results than some daffy diets, but the weight stays off, and your time is well spent by adapting and learning how to live with a new lifestyle that will last.

This method of slimming has four particular aspects:

1 Thinking: Think Slim is the key to slim-fit success.
2 WOW eating: Wise Or Wonderful eating, for nourishment and enjoyment.
3 Exercising that is kind, toning and energising.
4 Relaxing that is revitalising and motivating.

It's a pleasant way of transforming your fat life to a slim-fit one, *forever*.

Included are other stories of Think Slimmers who have succeeded too (see pages 235–241); and then a brief explanation of why it's necessary to drop out of the diet trap to start winning at slimming.

# DROPPING OUT OF THE DIET TRAP AND WINNING AT SLIMMING

## THE DIET TRAP

Diets don't work, partly because they begin on Monday – next Monday. Even before they start, we grant ourselves one last feast, stuffing in all our favourite food rather like the way the ancient Christians feasted richly on Shrove Tuesday before Lent began.

Then, when diets begin, they are soon broken: in a few days, a couple of hours or even 10 minutes. We declare that we will make up for our lapses, tomorrow. But we all know that tomorrow never comes.

Also, 'real life' gets in the way of our dieting, and we don't know how to cope: Christmas, holidays, the pre-menstrual syndrome or the menopause; the baby's ill, the work deadline's ominously near, the washing machine's broken down, and the cat's been sick. You could murder a few slices of sponge cake, and you do – well, actually you eat them, which is rather more fattening – but no diet sheet helps you cope with any of those problems and that dreadful urge to binge.

Or, the rules are so strict that we, mere normal frail human beings, are bound to fail. Then, when we fail, we begin to feel powerless and useless: a victim, not only of our diet but of our life, instead of its lead character.

'I'm hopeless and useless!' we fume at ourselves. Our self-esteem plummets, and the biscuits come out to comfort us. If, much later and pounds heavier, we begin again, it is with even less confidence in our ability to diet successfully than before. So, the next diet is almost doomed to failure before it is begun.

Even if we succeed, with iron will and punitive self-control, to adhere to a Very Low Calorie Diet (under 600 calories per day) the weight we watched fall off so joyously returns in ever faster waves. This is because our body, seeing itself to be threatened with starvation, 'helpfully' lowers its metabolic rate (the rate at which it burns up the calories) to enable us to survive on less food. Then as soon as we begin to eat over 600 calories again, the body is still burning the calories slower, so we put on weight faster.

Diets teach us to be dependent, upon the Expert and upon The Diet, and we try (and often fail) to obey inhumane or pointless rules. A well-known slimming group had, in its early years, a rule that no tomatoes should be eaten after midday. This rule was never explained to its members, who were told that it was good enough for the leader to lose weight, so it was good enough for them. Obey! Yours is not to reason why. This is no way to treat adult human beings. Two still-overweight refugees from that group recently defected to a group I run, and told me that they liked my approach so much better.

'There, we weren't allowed to answer back!' declared one.

'It was like being at Infants School!' complained the other, 'and there were so many rules and regulations. You felt like breaking them just because they were there!'

So, rebellion sets in, and both rules and diets are broken.

There is an interesting book with a title that tells it all about dependency: *If You Meet the Buddha On the Road, Kill Him.* The author, Sheldon Kopp, a psychotherapist, argues, rightly, that if you meet the Wise One with all the answers to your problems, with his/her set of rules and regulations for your life – flee! No one except you can find the best way for you to live your life and cope with your problems. So it is with the Diet Experts, with their Diet Sheets and No Tomatoes After Midday.

A diet is like a straitjacket. Someone else designed it; its aim is to control and restrain us; it doesn't fit; it feels uncomfortable, often painful; repeatedly and rebelliously we try to wriggle free, even if only for a little while; and we are longing to burst out of it at the earliest possible moment. And we do.

And the main reason why diets don't work is that sooner or later we intend that they will end. (Probably sooner.) Then we go back to our 'normal' eating with a thankful sigh – and very soon resume our 'normal' excess weight.

## DROPPING OUT OF THE DIET TRAP

Most of us would be willing to drop out if we could believe that there is an alternative. There is.

Instead of all these diets and dependency, we need to learn to be in charge of ourselves, choosing for ourselves, learning to slim successfully while receiving only guidance and support from other sources – becoming a Self-empowered Slimmer.

Dropping out of the Diet Trap is begun by banishing the word 'diet' from your vocabulary and from your thoughts.

'I've been dieting all week' could be 'I've been slimming all week'.

'Isn't it a pointless change of words?' I'm asked.

It isn't pointless. It is important. Words are very powerful. I expect most of us, as children, chanted the words 'sticks and stones may break my bones, but words will never hurt me' in an effort to defend ourselves from cruel words. But the chant was not true, and we all know it. Words can, and do, hurt. Words are important. We think in words, and our thoughts determine our attitudes. Our attitudes play an important part in the success or failure of our slimming.

'Anyone here on a diet?' I frequently yell out to my slimming group.

'No, no, no!' they shout in laughing response.

'Great!' I call back in praise, and if there is a newcomer, she/he is quite bemused by it all. She/he thought they came to a slimming group to be put on a diet. Diet is not a word that appears on any of the literature given to my group. Never say 'diet' again.

## START WINNING AT SLIMMING!

Instead of dwelling dismally in the straitjacket of the Diet Trap, we need to start slimming, which can be compared to making ourselves a made-to-measure dress. To dressmake, we purchase a good quality basic pattern, take heed of reputable advice, check our personal body requirements, amend the basic pattern to fit us, and start sewing. It takes a long time, effort and patience, but eventually it's worth it because we have something that fits and is as individual as we are.

So, I am no Diet Guru with List of Instructions for your life. I am trying to help you set yourself free; to empower you to empower yourself, to enable you to find the slim-answers to the unique slimming problems in your life. We need to think of ourselves as powerful, for we are. The self-empowered person is one who takes charge of his/her life; who diagnoses problems, and then seeks solutions or ways to cope; who lives life to the full. A self-empowered slimmer takes these principles and applies them to slimming. Step 1 of this programme, 'Empower Yourself' (the next chapter), explains more fully about being self-empowered.

An honest review of yourself and your lifestyle is needed. Then the secret of successful slimming lies in altering how you cope with your problems by changing how you think.

## DIET-THINK

Another destructive characteristic of dieting is that it is doomed by Diet-Think:

'I'll not have *any* chocolate, or alcohol, or cake . . .' we resolve, impractically.

'This dieting is so miserable,' we sigh, dejectedly.

'It's so Unfair!' we declare, miserably.

'Just this little bit won't hurt,' we kid ourselves, stupidly.

'Is that *all* I've lost?' we shriek, impatiently.

'It's just *not* worth it,' we conclude, finally.

All of these thoughts are destructive to our slimming efforts. Sometimes we don't even notice the thoughts, just our dejected mood. So what, you say?

The good news is that we can learn how to replace such destructive thoughts with more encouraging ones. Thinking comes naturally, for we are born with the capacity to think, but how and what we think is not natural, it is learned. We can learn to change it.

So, to summarise: to become slim and stay slim we need to drop out of the diet trap to become a self-empowered slimmer who replaces dieting with slimming, and Diet-think with Slim Think.

# PART I
# THE SEVEN STEPS TO SLIM-FITNESS

# EMPOWER YOURSELF!
## Think Slim –
## whose thoughts are
## they anyway?

Fourteen formidable stones of heaving green knitwear faced me. (That's 87½ kilos to you metric thinkers.)

'I've been to 12 slimming groups and the hypnotist and they've all failed and now I've come to see what *you* can do,' she declared decisively.

I smiled gently back at her. 'Oh no,' I replied softly, 'now we need to see what *you* can do.'

Jane was no Plain variety: pretty face, beautifully decorated; clothes well-matched and colour co-ordinated; but her potential elegance was spoiled by her overflow of flesh. She, clearly, felt resentful.

'I don't need anybody else to tell me that it's all *my* fault,' she began. 'I know that well enough already.'

I could understand how she felt. Others, and she herself, had been heaping blame upon her for years because she could not stick to their diets.

'I wouldn't dream of telling you it's your fault,' I said. 'I shall tell you that it's your responsibility, and your choice, but that's quite a different matter. No more blame. No more guilt.'

## BEING SELF-EMPOWERED

For many slimmers, life is something that happens to them while they comfort themselves with another biscuit. To be successful at slimming they need to use their thoughts to become self-empowered. Instead of asking what the Expert can do about their slimming, they need to see what they can do.

Successful people are self-empowered people. By 'successful' I do not mean that they are necessarily rich, famous or powerful – although they might be. By 'successful' I mean that they are living how they want to be living, in a positive way, while respecting themselves and others. They are not 'having it all', for that is a pipe dream, and choosing to do one thing often involves choosing not to do another; but they have what they have decided is more important to them; they are making the most of their lives. If the world is a stage, they are the producers, directors and lead characters in their own play.

In the film *Shirley Valentine*, Shirley, a hapless housewife, muses: 'I have led such a little life. I have allowed myself to lead such a little life.' Then she takes charge of her life (and if you haven't seen the film, dash to the video shop, soon). If, like Shirley, the only thing big about your life is your hip size, you need to become self-empowered.

While Disastrous Dieters let it happen, Successful Slimmers *make* it happen.

## THE MYTH: BORN TO BE . . .

'I've always been big. I must have been born to be big!' Caroline moans, prodding unhappily at her fleshy hips.

We are all born with certain characteristics – our eye colour, our height, perhaps some congenital disease, or handicap. Some people have unique talents: for music or artistry, athleticism, practicality, or academic genius. Our basic body shape (for example the female, 'pear'/ curvy/athletic/boyish; or the male, short and slight/tall and narrow/ broad/squat) are also predetermined. That predetermined shape can be padded with fat or not, depending on what we do. Our basic metabolic rate may be slower or faster than the average, and that does affect how quickly we store fat. It does not, however, determine how overweight we are. Our eating habits and exercise levels do that. Caroline was not born to have over-fleshy hips. Her eating habits and (lack of) exercise caused that.

We are born rather like a canvas where just a few brush marks have already been made, but with plenty of scope to become what others encourage, and we choose.

There is an odd paradox; we are born both powerful yet powerless. Powerless, having to depend upon adults for our survival, for food, shelter, warmth, and affection. Powerful, with loud lusty cries and an insatiable curiosity, with great courage and an enthusiastic keenness to learn.

And learn we do: from our family, our friends, our teachers, our culture. We learn to be less powerful; some of us learn to be helpless. We learn to be a good girl or a brave boy, to be quiet, not to answer back, not to say 'no', to think first of others, eat up all our dinner, and be grateful.

## THE REALITY: PROGRAMMED TO BE . . .

'My mother's fat, my sisters are fat. It must run in the family,' explained Josephine, arriving with her surplus pounds flowing around her.

What 'runs in the family' are eating habits, thinking habits and attitudes to food, slimming and life. In this sense, yes, we can be 'programmed' to be overweight, as we learn to overeat and under-exercise.

Psychology studies suggest that we learn as children by imitating those around us, and through reward and punishment, learn what to do and what not to do. Some psychologists believe that as tiny children we learn the 'scripts' that we replay later, in our adult lives, mainly unaware of the 'programming' that underlies what we do.

But our programming does not doom us forever. If we stop to reflect on our ideas, our attitudes and our behaviour, we can choose to cast them off, and to change to ways of thinking and living that serve us better.

What did we learn about eating? 'Clear up your plate.' I realised that I was even delighted with my dog when she cleared up her plate!

'I never buy ice-cream for myself,' boasted Moyra at my slimming group, but added, 'but I often have to finish up my daughter's.'

The childhood message was strong: 'Don't waste food – think about the starving millions.' But the message is irrational. How can it help the starving millions if we over-eat and are overweight?

'Eat it all up for Mummy' may have been actual words said to you by your anxious parent who wanted you to be a healthy, strong toddler. Young children desperately want and need to please their parents (even if it seems sometimes to a harassed mum that it's not so!), and they often comply with such a request to eat, simply to please. Pleasing others can make us feel good. Unfortunately, years later, we can still get that good, warm feeling from eating that was fixed in our minds in childhood when we pleased Mum.

Also, our mothers, wanting to give love, gave us cake, and taught us to comfort eat. A sweet to take away the taste of the nasty medicine; pudding after we'd been good by eating up our greens. Food as reward. Food as celebration.

Alternatively, if we were naughty, our parents may have used denial of food as a punishment: 'Off to bed you go, without any supper.' Much later, we adults who cannot even remember the childhood incidents, still associate denial of food with punishment. So it can be hard for us as adults to say 'No' to our favourite fattening foods, if we unconsciously think of it as a punishment rather than of our own wise choice.

Or, the eating of sweet foods might have been made more valuable in our childish eyes when we were told: 'No pudding until you've eaten up your greens!' Psychology investigations of children and food have found that children soon get to dislike foods that are 'forced' upon them, mainly because they associate those foods with coercion.

What did they teach us about a woman's place? It's where everyone else wants her to be. What about anger? Unladylike! If our man treats us abysmally, it must be because we ask for it, or we deserve it, and if only we were better (and slimmer) he would be good to us. When Sue's husband worked late on their anniversary evening, she sat waiting, dressed to the ninety-nines, restaurant table booked. Waiting and getting angrier. She knew only one way to cope – eat. She ate a whole rich fruit cake before he arrived home. She would have done better to cascade the crumbled cake over him as he walked through the door.

And what did they teach us about a man's position? He must be the breadwinner. Compete. No freedom to choose part-time working for him, however much he might hate his job. The more money he makes, the more of a Real Man and a Success he is. If She wants a new expensive bike for each of the kids, or the latest Laura Ashley flounce, He must get the money, or be a failure as a man. His feelings? He is not allowed them – well, except anger and aggression which are encouraged: 'Stand up for yourself. Don't cry.' 'Be a New Man but Don't be a Wimp – but one woman's New Man may be another woman's Wimp. Confused? Don't complain!' 'Father children; pay to keep them; but don't dare expect custody if your marriage breaks down.' 'Resentful? You've no right. Some feminists say it's all you men's fault anyway.'

When all this programming has worked and he can't share his feelings with his partner or his mates, well, let him eat liquid calories at the pub to anaesthetise his stresses, give him a gargantuan gut, and heighten his blood pressure. That is, after he's finished eating Man-sized meals (loadsa meat and no cissie vegie stuff).

And if his heart gives up under all this pressure: 'Has he made provision to provide for his family financially?'

As children we learned, when we made mistakes, that we were stupid, useless, bad. It is hardly surprising that we started to blame others and to make excuses, in an effort to defend ourselves, when we failed to achieve something. We carry this defensiveness forward into adulthood, and, when we fail to be slim, we defend ourselves with excuses and push blame onto others.

However we should not blame our parents for how they 'programmed' us. They were doing the best they knew. They, too, had been programmed by their parents before them.

We can begin to break free of this programming if we first are prepared to recognise it.

'I've not been programmed by my parents,' objected Dave, strongly. Sorry if it's not news that you like. You. Me. All of us. By parents, by friends, by our culture. It was inevitable; we were too young to do anything else but be programmed.

I remember the day that I knew I was free. I threw half a chocolate bar into the waste bin, simply because I didn't want any more, and none of my companions wanted it. Yet their reaction was incredulous and critical! You would have thought that I had publicly thrown my knickers in the air.

However, from out of all this programming, we can, as adults, learn to become self-empowered, by rethinking.

What does it mean, to be self-empowered?

# THE SELF-EMPOWERED SLIMMER

Being self-empowered means taking responsibility for ourselves, and taking charge of our lives, of our place in the world, and of our slimming. We shall never have complete control of the world, for there are too many factors that we as individuals cannot control.

Despite that, if we are self-empowered there is always an alternative and we can always choose. This is not to say that we shall always like the alternatives before us. Maybe you think like Maisie:

'But I want to eat all the nice things I love *and* I want to be slim,' she sighed.

I know how she feels. I agree with her. However, what she wants is simply not possible.

There is, however, for us, a choice. Either we eat everything we fancy and be overweight, or we 'give up to get' – give up some of our favourite foods to get a slim-fit life. The choice is ours. I know which I prefer.

There is another choice within that choice. We decide whether we 'give up to get' with an accepting and cheerful attitude, or whether we make ourselves miserable, moaning about how dreadful life is, forcing us to make this undesirable choice. Life is, simply, more enjoyable if we accept that which cannot be changed with cheerful acceptance. It also pays to make friends with other cheerful people, those who lift not deaden your spirits.

So, what is a self-empowered slimmer? (For 'her' and 'she' also read 'his' and 'he'.)

- The self-empowered slimmer does not abdicate her responsibility for her slimming to someone else (for that saps her confidence and her power to change herself). But nor does she accept blame, criticism and put-downs – either from others, or from herself (for that, too, spoils her confidence).
- She accepts that she over-eats. That is not necessarily to say that she massively over-eats, or that she always eats more than a slimmer friend. It means, simply, that she eats more than her, unique body needs.
- She observes herself, to become aware of why and how she eats, and how she thinks – not so as to heap self-blame upon herself, but as a basis from which to change.
- She accepts herself as imperfect. She does not seek perfection (in her looks, her household, or her relationships).
- She values herself, as a unique and valuable individual, worth no more, but no less than other people.
- She has a sense of humour, and does not take herself too seriously.
- She asserts her own rights.

The Rights and Responsibilities of the self-empowered slimmer can be expressed as a Bill and a Declaration. These follow, overleaf.

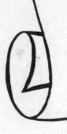

# THE SELF-EMPOWERED SLIMMER'S BILL OF RIGHTS

1   *I have the right to choose.*
2   *I am entitled to eat what I choose.*
3   *I have the right to take as long as it needs to slim.*
4   *I have the right to say 'No' to others.*
5   *I have the right to disagree.*
6   *I have the right to 'Me-time'.*
7   *I am entitled to regard myself as important – equally as important as other adults.*
8   *I have the right to regard my slimming as important.*
9   *I have a right to my feelings.*
10   *I have a right to ask for support and help.*
11   *I have the right to make mistakes.*
12   *I have the right to change.*
13   *I have the right to change my life for the better, for me.*

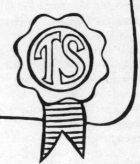

## RIGHTS: IN PRACTICE

Ideas are useful only when they lead to action. The Bill of Rights will help the slimmer to succeed if the ideas are put into practice. Following are examples of ways that the rights may affect slimmers.

### 1  I HAVE THE RIGHT TO CHOOSE

About my weight, my work, my life.

I can choose to settle for a Target Weight that suits me (as long as it's high enough to be healthy), rather than the one that is imposed by any Weight/Height Table, or by a slimming group leader.

I can choose to take a job, leave a job, or stay at home, rather than be dictated to by my family or society's ideas of what I should do (although I will take other people's opinions into account). It is my life, and I must decide what is best for me.

For example, Jenny, over 50, lost over five stones/31 kilos and got a job, for the first time in her long-married life; she learned to dance and do aerobics. 'I didn't know what I was missing!' she now declares.

## 2 I AM ENTITLED TO EAT WHAT I CHOOSE

I shall not allow others to put me down for eating my *moderate* chocolate, cake or other treats that I have chosen as part of my slimming strategy.

Babs reached her Target Weight while still enjoying a brandy every evening; Patsy's daily choice was a small chocolate bar.

## 3 I HAVE THE RIGHT TO TAKE AS LONG AS I NEED TO SLIM

I am a unique individual. No two people's bodies work exactly the same; no two people's lifestyles, needs and desires are exactly the same. I have the right to choose how many (or few) sacrifices I want to make, at any one time, in order to lose weight.

I don't compete with others in the Speedy Weight-Loss Game. I have no need to feel inadequate if it takes me longer to lose weight than it takes others.

Weight is gained over a long period of time and takes an even longer period to be (safely) shed. I may not like it, but that is Nature's law and beyond my control. I accept it, and others have no right to criticise how long it takes me to lose weight.

## 4 I HAVE THE RIGHT TO SAY 'NO' TO OTHERS

'No' to Mother-in-law who puts roast potatoes on my plate, or to Mum or friends who insist 'have a piece of cake, I made it especially for you'. 'No' to young children who thrust their toffees towards my mouth. 'No' to those who expect me to be their servant.

'No' to demands on my time, my patience, and my goodwill, when I believe that I have done enough.

## 5 I HAVE THE RIGHT TO DISAGREE

If I have a different view, I have a right to keep it.

'You should give up this dieting! You're already too thin!' plagues many a still-chubby-cheeked slimmer. I don't have to convince others I'm right. I can agree to disagree, and show them I'm right by the new slim-fit and healthy me.

## 6 I HAVE THE RIGHT TO 'ME-TIME'

Everyone has a right to 'me-time'. It is not cruelly self-centred – it is showing as much respect for myself as I show to others. Besides, I will be able to care better for those who need caring for in my life, when I feel fitter and more willing, having taken my 'me-time'.

## 7 I AM ENTITLED TO REGARD MYSELF AS IMPORTANT – EQUALLY AS IMPORTANT AS OTHER ADULTS

Equality is a basic human right. It doesn't mean, if you're a woman, that you have to burn your bra and stomp stridently about demanding a job as a coal-miner.

I regard myself as an 'equalist': one who accepts equal rights (and responsibilities) for all adults, whatever sex, colour, race, or age. Therefore the needs and wants of my mother/father/husband/wife/family are only *equally* as important as my own.

## 8 I HAVE THE RIGHT TO REGARD MY SLIMMING AS IMPORTANT

The plans, the shopping, the preparing of my slimming strategies are important, and need to be given higher priority than the dusting. (Your visitors should come to see *you*, not to check on your credentials for getting a job as Housekeeper at Buckingham Palace. If your partner is a house-proud perfectionist, that's his/her problem. Life's too short to spend it dusting. If you are slim enough, fit enough and lively enough, you and your partner will be too busy enjoying yourselves to fret and fuss about the dust.)

## 9 I HAVE A RIGHT TO MY FEELINGS

I am entitled to the whole range of my feelings. I do not have to suppress some because they are not ladylike, or macho, or popular. I am entitled to feel angry when it is justified, and to express that anger appropriately.

## 10 I HAVE A RIGHT TO ASK FOR SUPPORT AND HELP

I do not need to feel guilty about asking for help/support. We are only human, and learning to change your self and your life to slim is a difficult process. We succeed best with encouragement and support. Others cannot 'mind read', and may not be aware that we need support. So, it's necessary to ask for it.

## 11 I HAVE A RIGHT TO MAKE MISTAKES

. . . without being chastised by others or by myself as useless or hopeless. If I have 'failing days' when I give in to the temptation to over-eat, that means no more than that I am only human. I shall start better habits with determination.

## 12 I HAVE THE RIGHT TO CHANGE

There may be people in my life who don't want me to change. They are comfortable with me as 'good old Big Brenda'. I have no need to stay as uncomfortable as I am just because it suits others.

## 13 I HAVE THE RIGHT TO CHANGE MY LIFE FOR THE BETTER, FOR ME

The changes I make may involve more than just changes in my eating habits, but they will be for the better, for me. This is my life. This is not a rehearsal, and I am entitled to change it for the better, for myself.

---

# THE SELF-EMPOWERED SLIMMER'S DECLARATION OF RESPONSIBILITIES

*1 I am Responsible for myself, my weight, my slimming, and my life.*
*2 I am Responsible for my thoughts, feelings, and actions.*
*3 I am Responsible for respecting myself and others.*

---

## RESPONSIBILITIES: IN PRACTICE

Hand in hand with rights always go responsibilities. Accepting responsibility can seem burdensome sometimes, but it is something that can actually help the slimmer by aiding him/her to think honestly and realistically, paving the way for slimming success. Ways that responsibilities may affect slimmers follow.

### 1 I AM RESPONSIBLE FOR MYSELF, MY WEIGHT, MY SLIMMING AND MY LIFE

I do not blame others for my mistakes or misfortunes. NO excuses.

We are overweight because we over-eat (for our particular body and level of exercise).

I do not blame my excess weight on 'big bones' or other spurious notions.

No more excuses for sabotaging our slimming: 'It's his fault I ate that cake, because he was late and I was furious.' Fury in such a situation may be helpful. Eating isn't. Nor are excuses.

However, although I am responsible for my mistakes, I do not 'blame' and chastise myself for my mistakes. I am allowed to make mistakes. It is OK to be imperfect. I notice my mistakes, and plan how to avoid them again, then take action to do so. I do *not* continue to repeat my mistakes.

If my life is boring, or unsatisfactory, it's up to me to do something to change things.

### 2 I AM RESPONSIBLE FOR MY THOUGHTS, FEELINGS AND ACTIONS

It is not unusual to be seen as responsible for our actions, but we are also responsible for our thoughts and our feelings.

'Surely not!' you protest. '*He* made me angry!' Not actually so. He did something. You made yourself angry about it by the thoughts you chose. Maybe that was appropriate – to be angry can be useful. Florence Nightingale became angry, thinking about the conditions of hospitals, but she didn't sit fuming and chomping cake, she thought of ways to change things.

For women, and men, who are angry about the inconsiderate way their partner treats them, anger can be a useful fuel for demanding improvement – or leaving.

## 3 I AM RESPONSIBLE FOR RESPECTING MYSELF AND OTHERS

Everyone (including me) is entitled to respect. Yet it is I who am responsible for respecting myself and ensuring, as far as possible, that others respect me. For example, leaving work on time is a sign of respect for ourselves and our private life. Getting work done on time (without slacking) is respecting the boss and also our work-selves.

Losing excess weight is respecting oneself. Not stuffing our body with high-fat, high-sugar foods that punish our bodies, is a sign of respect for our physical self. So is giving nourishing food to our bodies. Looking slim and good is respecting our own wishes.

# ASSERT YOURSELF

These rights and responsibilities of the self-empowered slimmer follow the principles of assertiveness. Assertiveness is a particular way of thinking and of behaving.

Thinking assertively means believing that our own feelings, needs and wants are as important as those of other people.

Behaving assertively means choosing to act in accordance with that thinking. A person who is assertive practises what he/she preaches.

## THINKING AND ACTING ASSERTIVELY MEANS:

- Being honest with yourself, acknowledging your own feelings, needs and wants.
- Respecting yourself, that is, believing that you are equally as important as other people. Your feelings, needs and wants, therefore, are equally as important as theirs.
- Being honest in telling others about your feelings, needs and wants, in a considerate not aggressive manner, and without getting side-tracked. So you stand up for your rights without violating the rights of others.
- Accepting responsibility for yourself (your thinking, your feelings and your behaviour).
- Being able to give and receive compliments and constructive criticism.
- Being able to acknowledge and deal with your own anger in a constructive way.
- Being relaxed, comfortable and confident about these ways of thinking and behaving.
- The person who is assertive speaks confidently, says how she/he feels, and may use phrases such as:
  'What I would like is . . .'

'Would you please . . .?'
'What I should like you to do is . . .'
'No, I'm sorry, I cannot possibly . . .'
'I disagree. I think . . .'
'I didn't understand that; would you tell me again please?'
'I feel angry when you . . .'
'I feel taken for granted because . . .'
'I feel really pleased that . . .'

## THE ALTERNATIVE WAYS OF THINKING AND BEHAVING:

If you are not thinking and behaving assertively, you will be adopting one or a combination of the following styles:
- aggressive
- submissive
- passive
- manipulative

**The Aggressive** way is 'over the top'. Mr/Ms Angry are shouting, insulting, blaming, patronising and pushing their way through life. Ask them for a favour and they'll yell that 'you must be joking'. They dominate: 'It's no use you going to a slimming group, it's a waste of time and money.' Their wishes are almost always more important than yours. They are contemptuous, sarcastic, controlling, in either loud or quiet ways; sometimes even without words, but with a raised eyebrow, a contemptuous toss of the head, a sneering smirk or an aggressive or superior stance.

They may resort to violence to resolve their disagreements. They are Number One and everyone else must be lower in their pecking order. Equality is a dirty word. To them, Revenge is sweet, relationships are a power struggle, and life is a fairly nasty brutish business.

**The Submissive** style means going through life with a 'pardon me for living' approach. Someone treads on *her* toe and it is *she* who says sorry. She doesn't even ask for favours, for she expects none. She often says 'I'll do what you want' or 'you choose'. Her sentences frequently begin: 'This might sound silly but . . .' or 'I may be wrong but . . .'; 'I'm afraid I . . .', 'I wonder if you could possibly . . .'

Often a doormat, she wonders why people walk all over her when she is simply trying so hard to be nice. She thinks that perhaps if only she tries harder to be nicer, perhaps they'll be nicer and she'll get her just rewards. Fat chance!

**The Passive** approach involves standing back and letting life happen to you. The passive person never initiates: where to go, what to do, what to buy, and never makes the first move in love-making.

If asked to choose, these folk reply 'I don't mind'. If decisions are to be made, they mutter: 'well, I'll wait and see what happens . . .' Nothing is ever his/her fault (and that can have an advantage because it can feel quite comfortable). Similar to the submissive, Mr/Ms Passive are not in the director's seat in their own life; they have walk-on parts and act out someone else's script.

**The Manipulative** manner means getting your own way by stealth. The Manipulators' relationships are not honest, for they are busily pretending to be nice guys while working to getcha. Then they are secretly pleased with their own 'cleverness'. But they are not clever enough to see that they miss out on the better benefits of relationships based on honesty. They may offer you choices, but they are 'weighted' to the result they really want. ('Would you like to go shopping? We can, but it'll be very crowded, and tiring. I don't know where we'll park the car. We've got to be back early, and we're very overspent this month . . .')

Their energies are used up in continuous plotting. When they fail, they feel frustrated, and that frustration festers, hidden too.

The passive, submissive and manipulative styles may well eventually break out into violent aggression, or into binge-eating to relieve the tension. Often, overweight people are those who have been conditioned by their upbringing into being 'too kind for their own good'. Although such people feel that they must put others' needs before their own, frustrations build up and are often 'eaten away' rather than expressed appropriately.

Alternatively, as Jacqui explained: 'When I get very fat, I feel as if I have to be extra nice to people, and do what they want me to, as if I have to make up for being so fat. Then I get fed up with being put upon, but I just eat my way through it . . .' Jacqui would be happier and slimmer if she chose to be assertive about her needs and wants.

If your anger and frustrations are stuffed down with food, don't continue to suffer, swallowing your feelings with food and spoiling your slimming. You need to express yourself, clearly, politely and firmly to all around you.

Assertiveness is for both women and men. Often, it is women who suffer from being unassertive, due to their 'be-a-good-little-girl' upbringing. Some men, who as boys learned far too well to 'stand up for themselves' are too aggressive and need to replace that aggression with assertion. Other men suffer, as do many women, from being unassertive, but may break out, when under pressure, into a destructive burst of violence. Assertiveness is the moderate and positive way.

The more assertive we are, the less aggressive we are likely to be, as aggression is often fuelled by anger and frustration at not being treated equally and not getting our own needs and wants met reasonably often enough.

Being assertive does not guarantee that we will always get our own way, and we need to respect the rights of others to have different wants from ourselves. However, if we act assertively, we are more likely to get what we want more often, so that when we don't, we can be happier to compromise.

Acting assertively is a skill which, like any other, needs to be practised. In time, it becomes easier. The more you do it, the more confident you become, and just as 'vicious circles of behaviour can become an undermining habit, so a 'successful' circle of assertiveness can develop which can positively help you. It goes like this:

## THE SUCCESSFUL CIRCLE OF ASSERTIVENESS

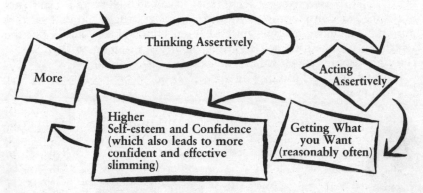

### TEACHING YOURSELF ASSERTIVENESS
Re-read this section often, so that you get to feel comfortable with the ideas, and take time to think about your own approach to your life. You could begin by considering, on a scale of 0–10, how assertively you think and act, generally, in your life.

| 0 | 1 | 2 | 3 | 4 | 5 | 6 | 7 | 8 | 9 | 10 |
|---|---|---|---|---|---|---|---|---|---|---|

0=Unassertive                                       10=Confidently Assertive

Then consider which of the alternative styles – passive, submissive, manipulative, or aggressive – best describes your behaviour. Many people operate differently in different situations: for example, at work, with parents, with spouse or partner, with adult children, or with friends.

Think about when you think and behave unassertively (and maybe afterwards, reach for the biscuits): with which people? In which situations? Consider how you could handle them more assertively.

Try being assertive. Try, first, in situations which seem easiest for you. Experiment. Practise what you want to say, in advance. Don't worry that this seems artificial. You'd be surprised how many confident 'off the cuff' remarks of others have been well rehearsed beforehand. Refer back to the assertive 'start-phrases' outlined at the beginning of this section; learn and use them to help you to express yourself until you are more confident.

Even if, by being assertive, you don't always get what you want, you'll usually feel better for having had your say, and are less likely to get the urge to chomp at cheesey chunks in frustration.

If you'd like further help, there are books you can read about assertiveness (see Further Reading, page 275) and you may well find part-time assertiveness courses advertised in your area.

## ASSERTING YOURSELF – DOUBTS!

Some slimmers have 'doubts'. One, in particular, goes something like: 'doesn't all this assertiveness mean that I'm selfish?' Not at all. The rights give you *equal* consideration with others. It is not suggested that you are more important than others, just of equal importance. That is not the 'selfishness' or the total self-centred-'I'm-all-Right-Jack-and-Bunnies-to-You!' philosophy which we are, rightly, taught to avoid.

'I felt guilty! I'd disappointed her!' said Patsy, speaking of her demanding mother.

'That's OK' I reassure her.

'OK?!!!!' she screeched. For Patsy, as for many of us, it is almost heresy to say that it's OK to disappoint important people in our lives. That is how many women have been conditioned to think all their lives. From being little, good girls, they go on as adults, still trying to be good girls, but failing to be good enough, and eating fruit cake to stem their anxiety or to quieten their guilt. It is unproductive. It makes us unhappy and overweight.

If others make what you feel are unreasonable demands on you, you are entitled to 'disappoint' them. We are entitled to what has been called 'enlightened self-interest'.

## ASSERTIVENESS: IN PRACTICE

Putting the assertiveness, rights and responsibilities into practice will help you to slim. However, the examples given in the preceding pages do not, of course, cover all situations that a slimmer will find her/himself in. But you will be able to apply the principles to any situation that faces you.

At first, it may be somewhat difficult to apply the principles consistently. That's not unusual when we are trying something new: applying new ideas, or applying new skills. So persevere, and it will become easier.

Follow this process:
- Thoroughly read this section, The Self-Empowered Slimmer, pages 17–47.
- Re-read it often.
- As you read, consider situations in your life where the principles can apply.
- Think in advance how you might tackle a situation for yourself.

- Think before you act, or eat, or reply to someone.
- Review what you did. Could you have done it more usefully?
- Learn from your review. Plan for another time.
- Create your own Think Slim answers or strategies. Write them down; learn them, and review them. You could use the space below:

...........................................................................................................................

...........................................................................................................................

...........................................................................................................................

...........................................................................................................................

...........................................................................................................................

...........................................................................................................................

# THINKING ABOUT YOUR THINKING

Diets have always been based on the psychological theories of Behaviour Modification: instructions, rewards, and punishments are given. Eureka! – behaviour is changed. Behaviour Modification was investigated in laboratories with rats. It works well with rats, but people are more complicated (thank goodness!).

The great philosopher, Descartes, declared: 'I think, therefore I am.' He said that the essence of being human is that we can think about our own thinking (unlike animals, who can't).

Thinking happens in the brain as a result of what we see and sense around us. The brain does not work like a camera, reflecting the world as it is exactly; the brain interprets what we see and sense.

Psychologists have used the picture overleaf to demonstrate how our brain can interpret in more than one way. Look at the picture. What do you see? An old ugly crone? A young beautiful woman? Can you see first one, then the other? (It is not possible to see them both together, although you may be so fast at changing from one to the other that it seems as if you can. That illustrates the speed of your thought-processes.)

This picture demonstrates that it is our thoughts that interpret the world around us. Our interpretation of what we see is affected by our previous experiences, by what we expect to see, and what we are interested in seeing. We can continue seeing our world in the same old predictable way: maybe with over-rosy spectacles, or through dark depressing glass, or with unrealistic or romantic expectations. Or, we can decide to see what we want to see. We can decide to adopt what attitudes we want to adopt.

Thoughts often arise, apparently unbidden and uninvited. Then they influence how we feel. But it is possible to 'catch the thought', monitor what we are thinking, and then, consciously and deliberately, think about those thoughts.

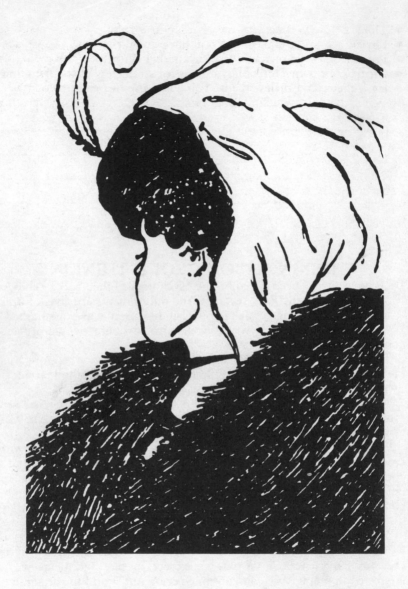

Why is it necessary to examine our thoughts? It is because thoughts have very powerful effects on our lives.

## THE POWER OF THOUGHT

If you were asked to walk along a plank about 12 inches/30 centimetres in width, placed on the floor, you would have no problem with the task.

Now, if you were asked to perform the same task, when the plank was placed 20 feet/6 metres up in the air, would you have a problem? Of course. The task is the same – to walk along the plank. The plank is no smaller in width. The difference is in what you think about the task.

Try a little experiment, right now. Imagine that you are picking up an orange . . . imagine you are peeling it . . . peeling back the bright orange skin. See the white-ish skin beneath . . . and you are going to bite into it. Bite it . . . and notice its tangy sweetness, its juiciness . . . Now, notice your mouth. Has there been a real change in your saliva? Your thoughts and your imagination are powerful.

Kate is an intelligent, capable woman who came to ask my help for her problem of agoraphobia.

'When I'm shopping in a department store,' she explained, 'I just start to feel panicky. I can hardly breathe, I start to gasp for breath, and I feel my heart going bump-bump-bump. It's awful, and I think I'm going to collapse. I just have to rush out.'

She was suffering from physical panic attacks that were triggered by something in her thoughts. The physical symptoms escalated as her thoughts became more frantic. She may well have caused herself to collapse, if she had continued to think 'panic-thoughts' which caused her over-breathing.

Instead, Kate learned how to catch the trigger-thoughts that started her attacks, and learned to replace them with calm-thoughts; she conquered her physical problem by the use of her thinking.

Medicine is full of stories to indicate the power of the mind (ie, our thoughts) over our physical body. A mother, desperate to save her trapped child, is capable of lifting weight that never, before or after, she could achieve.

Carl and Stephanie Simonton, in their book *Getting Well Again*, tell of cancer patients at their centre in Dallas, Texas, who, despite a terminally ill prognosis, continued to survive their illness. Dr Simonton teaches patients to use their minds to strengthen their body's natural defence system to fight the illness. They use the power of thought, through relaxation and imagination.

Our actions are either trapped into failure – or set free to succeed – by our thoughts.

# SLIMMING AND THINKING

We can harness all this thought-power so that we can succeed with our slimming.

In the past, you have lived with thought-habits that have hindered your attempts at losing weight, and yet you have not even been aware that thought-habits played a part.

Let's consider the way that we have failed on diets, before. It is illustrated by the following diagram: The Vicious Circle of Diet Failure.

# THE VICIOUS CIRCLE OF DIET FAILURE

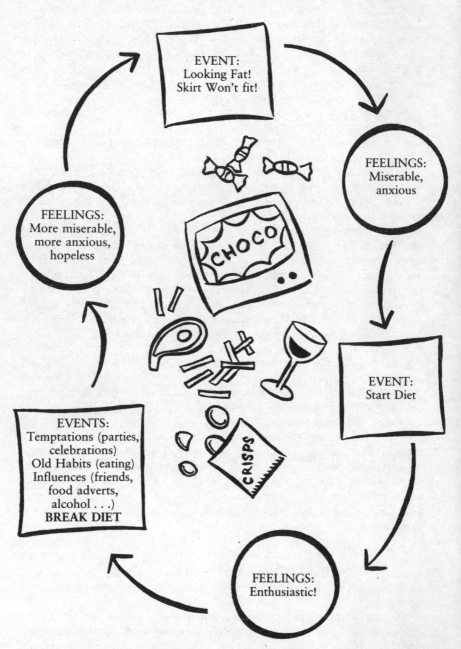

EVENT:
Looking Fat!
Skirt Won't fit!

FEELINGS:
Miserable,
anxious

FEELINGS:
More miserable,
more anxious,
hopeless

EVENT:
Start Diet

EVENTS:
Temptations (parties,
celebrations)
Old Habits (eating)
Influences (friends,
food adverts,
alcohol . . .)
**BREAK DIET**

FEELINGS:
Enthusiastic!

## *THE VICIOUS CIRCLE OF DIET FAILURE – AND HOW TO BREAK IT*

Are you only too familiar with that vicious circle? Certainly, I remember it well. For fifteen years I was in its grip, my weight yo-yoing up and down, depending where I was on the circle. From size 10 to size 16. (And remember that I am only 4 feet 10 and three quarter inches (1½ metres) tall, so size 16, for me, is extremely round.) I felt as if I was doomed to spin, powerless, round and round: fatter, thinner, fatter . . . miserable, brighter, miserable. It feels truly vicious, that circle.

Then, finally, I found how it is possible to break it. From my studies of psychology, I learned that the circle, as illustrated, misses out something very important – our thoughts. This is a crucial factor for slimmers, and I shall tell you how to make use of it shortly.

Our feelings are *not* caused by events, but by our *thoughts about* those events.

## THE *COMPLETE* VICIOUS CIRCLE OF DIET FAILURE – AND HOW TO BREAK IT

The complete circle (overleaf) shows the part played by our thoughts in our attempts to lose weight.

Every minute of the day our thoughts race on, mostly without us being consciously aware of it. Your thoughts create a sort of running commentary of what's going on around you in your life. You can check this out by taking a minute or so just to stop reading this book, and to let your mind wander, while you 'listen' to your wandering thoughts. All day, your thoughts are never still.

Some psychologists have described this phenomenon as 'the chatter-box' in our head. It's not only the insane who talk to themselves! (The difference between the normal person with the 'chatterbox' thoughts and those who are mentally ill and 'hear voices' is that the mentally ill perceive the 'voices' as outside themselves, as real separate entities who control them from 'out there'.)

I'm sure that you can now recognise this complete vicious circle, and understand how your thoughts play a part. The thoughts are often old thought-patterns, acquired without you being conscious of it, nor critically examining what you think.

# THE *COMPLETE* VICIOUS CIRCLE OF DIET FAILURE

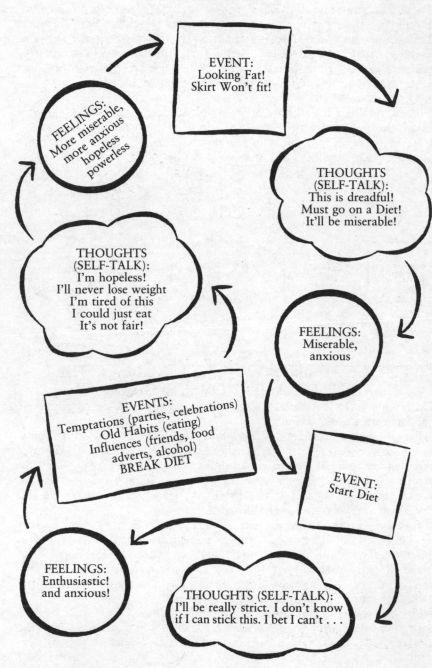

# BREAKING THE *COMPLETE* VICIOUS CIRCLE OF DIET FAILURE

**EVENT:**
Looking Fat!
Skirt Won't fit!

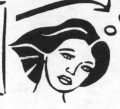

**THOUGHTS (SELF-TALK)**
I don't want this.
I will start slimming.
I will persevere
I know it will take a long time,
and that's OK.

**FEELINGS:**
Capable,
confident,
optimistic

**EVENT:**
Make plans,
start slimming

**THOUGHTS (SELF-TALK):**
I'll include some of my favourite foods
I'll aim to lose the first half stone/3 kilos
If I slip up, never mind – get back on track

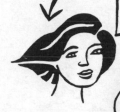

**EVENTS**
Temptations (parties, celebrations)
Old Habits (eating)
Negative Influences (friends, food
adverts, alcohol)
**DO NOT BREAK DIET:**
Sometimes resist;
other times, over-indulge.

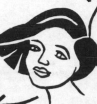

**FEELINGS:**
Capable,
confident,
optimistic

**THOUGHTS
(SELF-TALK):**
I blew it there,
but that's OK,
nobody's perfect
Back on track
now . . .
it's no disaster

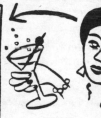

**FEELINGS:**
Coping –
doing OK
Confident,
optimistic

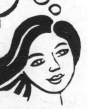

**EVENT:**
See less fat, weigh
less.
Skirt almost fits
Continuing –
to Slim-self

It is possible to break the vicious circle by

1 Making ourselves aware of the destructive thought-patterns.
2 Replacing them with more useful ones – 'Think Slim' thoughts.

'Think Slim' thoughts are crucial for slimming success to break the vicious circle of over-eating that ruins our slimming. Often, over-eating and bingeing are prompted by our feelings. And those feelings are prompted by our thoughts.

This is because our feelings are *not* really caused by events, but by our thoughts *about* those events. Our thoughts are often negative and depress our spirits; and 'Nega-think' for slimmers is often 'Fat-think' because they rush to eat cake for comfort. This is shown by the next diagram:

## NEGA-THINK TO THINK SLIM

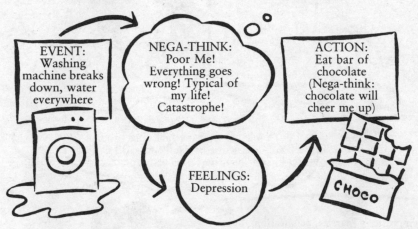

Now consider the same event, but with different thinking about that event, different feelings – and different outcome.

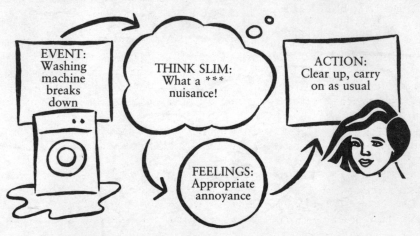

## COMPARING NEGA-THINK TO THINK SLIM:

Nega-think: 'Poor me.' 'Everything goes wrong!' 'Typical of my life!'

Nega-think is characterised by its negative, downbeat overtones. It suggests that life is against us; that we are unlucky; that we are helpless victims buffeted by whatever comes along; unable and incapable of doing what we want or achieving what we desire. It is unrealistic and 'over the top', because no one is actually as helpless as that. Nega-think makes mountains out of molehills, and suffers from 'can't-stand-it-itis'. Some psychologists have called this 'catastrophising' or 'awfulising'.

Recently I saw an interview on television with a professional entertainer famous mainly for her bulk, which audiences appear to find amusing. This roly-poly woman commented: 'Life must be awful if you can't eat everything you want.'

She was 'awfulising'; indulging in nega-think. I have news for her, and anyone else; life *isn't* awful when you can't eat everything you want. Life's too short to live it fat, and to compromise, so that you 'give up to get' (that is, give up some of the food you want, to get slim-fit) is making the most of your life. People who are the most deprived are those who deprive themselves of all the pleasures of being slim-fit.

So, nega-think makes the world and your life seem harder and blacker than it really is. Cherie Carter Scott, an American counsellor, suggests that some people are so trapped in this sort of thinking that they could be referred to as 'negaholics'. Fortunately, however, this sort of 'addiction' is not physical, and you can learn to change it.

Nega-think makes slimming tougher, and failure much more likely. It is the sort of thinking that keeps that old vicious circle of defeat going around. But it can be replaced by Think Slim.

## THINK SLIM IS REALISTIC

Notice the Think Slim which replaced the Nega-think in our example, where the washing machine broke down and there was water all over the floor: 'What a **** nuisance!' (Choose your own expletive.) Not that Think Slim is always a curse! However, in this case, a *realistic* thought-reaction would probably be something of that sort. Think Slim is realistic – not 'catastrophising'. If our thoughts are realistic then the feelings which follow will be realistic, not over-the-top, not causing the sort of stress that demands cake or chocolate to alleviate it. We stress ourselves by the thoughts we think. We de-stress ourselves by reshaping our thoughts.

Think Slim is realistic about a 'failed' day of slimming; it is not a catastrophe, merely a set-back, from which we can bounce back, and try again.

It is realistic, too, about how long it takes to slim. We all want to be slim yesterday, but to Think Slim is to recognise reality. Slimming takes a long time. We must cultivate perseverance. There is a sure-fire three-point basic plan for success: persevere, persevere, persevere.

## THINK SLIM IS POSITIVE

In the broken washing machine example, the next thought could be about how much time it would take to clear up. Nega-think would be estimating a whole week, and eating a bag of chips as consolation. Think Slim takes a positive view, and starts to clear up with a 'never mind, what can't be cured must be endured, let's get it over with' train of thought.

Think Slim is positive about slimming. It's not slimming that's miserable – being fat is. Slimming is solving a problem.

Think Slim is positive about ourselves. We forgive ourselves for our over-eating lapses and determine to do better. We begin to believe that we can 'do better', cultivating a 'can-do' positive attitude, but this must be allied to the realism mentioned above; it would be foolish to think that we 'can-do' the impossible, such as lose two stones/13 kilos by next week. 'Positive Thinking' ideas have sometimes had a bad press, deservedly so when they are presented as a magic wand to make things happen merely by thinking of them (like the 'I will win a fortune in a competition next Thursday' type of positive thinking). However, believing in ourselves is a very useful form of positive thinking.

Maria amazed her friends with her consistent, week-by-week weight losses. She explained: 'All I've done is stop thinking that I can't do it.'

Changing your negative can't-do thoughts to positive can-do thoughts frees you to succeed at slimming. It lifts your spirits, and you try harder.

There used to be a little eight-year-old boy-terror in my classroom, struggling to learn to read. He used to sigh, to me: 'But it's hard, Miss.'

I would reply: 'I know it's hard. But I know a really wonderful secret way to do something that's hard.' His eyes gleamed and his ears, for once, listened. 'When it's hard,' I whispered, 'you try harder.'

He laughed, but he tried harder, and he learned to read. Just as you can learn to slim and succeed. Slimming is hard, but it is possible, and we need to try hard, and harder, with a positive attitude.

Anna decided to slim after she had helped with a group of handicapped children on holiday. She said: 'They had so many handicaps. I thought, if they can manage to cope with their handicaps, and be cheerful, surely I can manage to slim and be cheerful.' Anna succeeded; she lost over two stones/13 kilos.

We slimmers need to do what the old song suggests and 'count our blessings'. Psychologists call it focusing on the positive. Look for the positive parts of your life and your slimming; focus on those, instead of dwelling on the dull, depressing bits. When you have lost a small amount of weight, don't moan that it's not enough; congratulate yourself, think delightedly that you are on the right track, and keep moving down that track.

## THINK SLIM IS HONEST

Think Slim avoids excuses. Excuses can't help you slim. Excuses leave you kidding yourself, stuck in a fat life that could be better.

Think Slim: we are overweight because we over-eat (for our individual body and our level of activity).

## THINK SLIM IS RATIONAL

Rational thinking means basing your thoughts on logic and reasonableness, sifting evidence and coming to rational conclusions.

The eminent Swiss psychologist, Piaget, investigated the stages in the development of thinking maturity. Young children use what he called 'concrete operational' thinking. That is, they can only grasp a few aspects of a problem, can describe but not logically explain them using abstract thought.

For example, young children need 'counters' or an abacus to help them to do arithmetic; they cannot yet use abstract logical thought. They may believe that things happen by 'magic', and attribute events as being caused by 'luck' or assume causes that are not rational. So, you may hear a child talking about his schoolwork, who says: 'I always get a good mark, then a bad mark, in English.' She or he, having believed that this is some fixed pattern outside his control, will unconsciously contrive to produce a good piece of work followed by a bad one, so making the pattern happen again.

During early adolescence, children's thinking should change in quality; they can handle more data, and use abstract logic. People vary as to when, or how well, they make this transition.

Many of us may use logical, rational thinking in the work areas of our lives, but not transfer it to our personal sphere. Many of our personal attitudes and our thinking about ourselves and our lives are also fixed irrationally from our upbringing – the 'programming' already discussed. So, instead of using rational thought, we simply continue in a way we have always done.

'That's me, I always eat when I'm stressed. You do, don't you?' declares many a harried slimmer. Certainly, many slimmers so deal with stress by eating, but it is not universal, nor inevitable. There are other ways of reacting to stress. The *que sera, sera* thinking habit is not rational thought. It is a 'programmed' habit.

We need to search our thinking habits for the automatic programmed thoughts from our upbringing and our families, test them for rationality, and replace them with rational logical thoughts that will help, not hinder, our slimming.

The famous psychologist, Eric Berne, suggested that as adults, we relive the patterns of behaviour he called scripts that we learned in childhood. Many of those behaviours are negative and destructive 'games' rather than honest, adult relationships. He labelled the styles of behaviour as those of 'Parent', 'Adult' and 'Child'. He created a diagram to illustrate his ideas, which looked something like this:

## PATTERNS OF THINKING AND BEHAVING
(After Eric Berne)

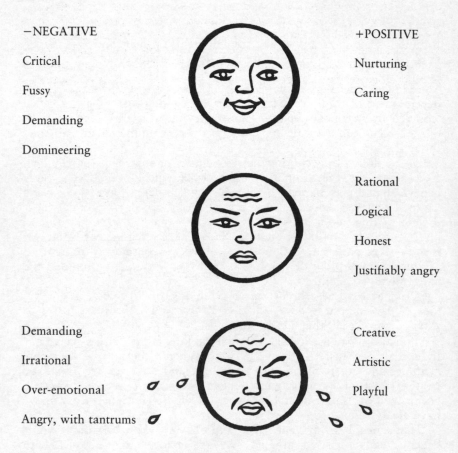

−NEGATIVE

Critical

Fussy

Demanding

Domineering

+POSITIVE

Nurturing

Caring

Rational

Logical

Honest

Justifiably angry

Demanding

Irrational

Over-emotional

Angry, with tantrums

Creative

Artistic

Playful

The Parent style can be positive, nurturing and caring (and that can include nurturing ourselves, into slim fit healthy beings). But it can also be negative: critical, domineering, hurtful, with many 'you shouldn'ts' and 'you can'ts' that undermine our confidence.

The Child pattern can be positive, creative, artistic, truly playful in a non-hurting way. But the child behaviours can also be destructive: 'I want, now' with impatience, and tantrums if thwarted.

The mature Adult style is rational, logical, honest; not manipulative nor exploiting.

Berne's ideas are useful for slimmers. We need to get rid of old behaviour and thought patterns. Behaviour patterns are prompted by swift, almost unnoticed, thought patterns. Think-slimmers need to avoid the Child's 'I want, now' demands, impatience, and tantrums; and to avoid the critical Parent thoughts such as 'I'm useless at slimming' and 'I can't succeed'. Instead, we need to rediscover our playful creative Child. Go to evening classes and paint or sculpt, hang-glide, garden, arrange flowers, dance or climb mountains; allow ourselves to be our own nurturing Parent, being kind to our bodies by eating healthy foods, resting when needed, pampering, relaxing. Especially, we need to adopt the rational style of thought of the mature adult: 'I might have failed at slimming before, but I'm going to improve now; I'm starting slimming with a wise eating plan; I'm contenting myself with small, healthy weight losses; I'm persevering to learn new eating habits; I'm planning and doing (such as exercise), not making excuses.'

To summarise: thought-power needs to be harnessed to help our slimming. The vicious circle of diet failure has been caused by old thought habits which have hindered our slimming efforts. To break this vicious circle, we change our thought patterns to Think Slim. Think Slim is realistic, positive and honest.

## THINK SLIM PROMPT CARDS

Throughout this book you are asked to make Think Slim Prompt Cards. The aim of this is to help you to re-programme those thought habits that have been destructive to your past efforts to slim.

The cards work when you repeat them often. Just as when you were a young child you learned the alphabet, the days of the week and the months of the year in order, by reciting them, so you can learn new thought patterns in a similar way. It is helpful to say the words aloud, and to tell them to other people (a slimming friend?).

This is based on the theory that we remember:
10 per cent of what we hear
30 per cent of what we see
50 per cent of what we see and hear
90 per cent of what we say.

Cut some thin card about 5 inches by 3 inches (13 cm by 8 cm); write big and bold, perhaps with felt pens.

It is also suggested that you create some Think Slim statements for yourself. When you do this, bear these points in mind:
1 The statement should be short.
2 It is easier to remember if it rhymes.
3 It should be written in the present, not future tense, eg 'I am successfully slimming' not 'I will be successfully slimming'. (Even if the statement does not quite ring true yet, do it this way, because it works best.)
4 It is better if the phrase is positive, eg 'I will/I am . . .' rather than 'I will not/I am not . . .'
Other ways to use your Think Slim Phrases:

Aileen had a white T-shirt printed with the phrase most helpful to her:
  Do I really want it?
  No, I don't.
  Shall I eat it?
  No, I won't!

You can also use Post-It notes, stuck in strategic places (on the biscuit tin, cupboards, mirror, or in the car). You could make posters with bright felt pens (teach yourself calligraphy, or go to a class). I have 'Do not distress yourself with Imaginings' on my study wall to rescue me from slipping into worry-thoughts. Or you could even embroider a cushion, or a wall hanging.

At the end of the book there is also a list of Think Slim Prompts for you to consult, or even photocopy if you wish. See page 271.
  When life in the fat lane is no longer enough, we can change ourselves from overweight to slim-fit by the process explained below.

# WHEN LIVING IN THE FAT LANE IS NO LONGER ENOUGH

YOUR OVERWEIGHT SELF:
Change Your Thoughts, from Diet-Think to Think Slim,
and become Self-empowered

Changes

Your Self-image and Your Self-esteem

Changes

Your Habits and Attitudes

Change to Slim-fit eating

Your slim and fit self

Diet-Think fails most because when we go on a diet, the regime is such a straitjacket — all cottage cheese and carrots and ne'er a chocolate in sight — that we intend to come off the diet as soon as possible. Which we do. Then we return to our 'normal' eating habits.

But it was our normal eating habits that led to our being overweight, so in no time at all we are overweight again. I call this the Sisyphus Syndrome; Sisyphus was, according to Greek legend, doomed to roll a great boulder up a hill, only to have it fall back each time to the bottom; then poor Sisyphus had to start his task all over again.

For dieters it can be worse, for often they put on more weight than before. This can happen especially if they lower their calorie intake to well under 1000 calories per day, because their body may well reserve its strength by lowering its Basal Metabolic Rate (BMR, the rate at which it burns calories). When the dieter resumes normal eating, the weight is regained, even faster, because the body has learned to use less calories than before. So, on/off dieting needs to be abandoned if the slimmer is to finally succeed.

The Key to slimming success is in changing our thoughts.

## THE WAY TO CHANGE OUR THOUGHTS

### 1 CATCH THE THOUGHT
First, we need to know what thoughts are reeling around in our head, spoiling our slimming. So, the first task is to 'catch the thought'. This means paying attention to your thoughts, and to the statements you make to others.

This is a new process and it may take some time to become adept at it. Persevere. Only when you are aware of your destructive thought patterns will you be able to replace them with more helpful ones. The next sections of this book will give you examples to start you off. Listen to other people's comments, about slimming and eating; spot their unhelpful nega-thoughts, and adopt any helpful ones you hear.

### 2 CHANGE THE THOUGHT
To change the thought, using the Thought-stopping Technique: simply say to yourself 'Stop!' and replace your unhelpful thought with your Think Slim replacement.

For example, she/he thinks:

| | |
|---|---|
| The Spoiler thought: ............... | 'I might as well eat it, that little bit won't hurt!' |
| Stop the thought: .................... | 'Stop!' |
| Change to Think Slim: ........... | 'Every little bit hurts. If it goes into my mouth it will settle on my hips! Shall I exercise it off? No. I just won't eat it.' |

## WHERE TO BEGIN: CHANGE 'DIET-THINK' TO 'THINK SLIM'

Firstly, replace Diet-Think with Think Slim: 'I'm *not* on a diet. I'm living the slim-fit lifestyle, forever.'

If that thought fills you with a moment's horror – 'what's this, a forever diet?!' – relax. Thinking Slim isn't like that, and I know because I'm a pleasure lover, and I've tried and succeeded with it; and when you read the food and drink programme (page 184) you will be even more reassured.

You need to banish the word diet from your thoughts, for if you think you are on a diet, you will be thinking about coming off it again. That's no help. You need a slim-fit lifestyle that will last for a lifetime.

To live the slim-fit lifestyle you need to be self-empowered, accepting responsibility for yourself, taking charge of yourself, your eating, your slimming and your life generally, using the principles already explained in the Self-empowered Slimmer's Bill of Rights and Declaration of Responsibilities.

These two changes will enhance your self-image and your self-esteem. That is necessary to help you succeed. Let's consider what is meant by self-image and self-esteem and how they affect the slimmer.

## SELF-IMAGE

'I'm a dieting disaster' were the first words Jill spoke to me, when she joined my group. Her unhappy 20-stone/125-kilo body seemed to prove that her self-image was right – that she was indeed a dieting disaster.

Our self-image is a mental picture that we hold of ourselves, of who and what we are. Jill believed that she was a dieting disaster; that she was a failure at losing weight. That thought was lodged firmly in her subconscious mind, and it ensured that she stayed that way.

Some young men choose to have 'born to lose' tattooed on their hands. It is also 'tattooed' on their brain, in their thoughts and in their subconscious mind, and they will surely lose at anything they attempt. They have programmed themselves to fail; they will never really put all their heart and soul into winning. So it is with slimmers.

Jill went on to change her thoughts, her eating habits and her body. The first thing Jill had to learn was to say and think: 'I *used to be* a dieting disaster.' She wrote this on a personal card, followed by the words: 'Now I'm a Successful Slimmer.'

What thoughts do you have about your image as a slimmer/dieter? If you have a problem similar to Jill's, tackle it the same way. Make a Think Slim card that tackles your problem and read and repeat the words in your thoughts, very often each day. Try to 'catch the thought' that keeps you fat, trapping you with a self image of failure.

'I've got no will-power!' is another counter-productive self-image description that is often repeated by slimmers. I joke with them; I can prove to them that they have will-power. You remember those occasions when you are out for a meal, have had a starter and a substantial main course? Your stomach's hunger is satisfied; you are feeling full. Then the sweet trolley arrives, groaning with tempting goodies. Yes, you bravely summon up loadsa will-power, and you are determined to eat that sweet, even if you can't move out of your chair afterwards! Such strong will-power you possess!

Such a situation proves, not that you have will-power, but the power of motivation. (You can read more about motivation in Step 3, page 117.)

Slimmers speak of will-power as if some people 'have it', as if it exists, like blue eyes. It doesn't. Pathologists, cutting up bodies and brains for a hundred years, have never found a section of the human body that is 'will-power'. There is a speech centre in the brain, along with vision and hearing points; there is a control centre for hormonal activity. There is nothing that can be labelled will-power. The notion of will-power – which we possess or don't – is an irrational Old Wives Tale (probably from a fat old wife who wanted an excuse for her bulk!). Forget the very idea of will-power. Stop using or thinking the words. Banish them forever. If the thought comes to you, use the Thought-stopping Technique.

Alternatively, perhaps you were raised in a family where chubbiness was praised; perhaps a beloved Grandpa nicknamed you 'cuddles' or told you lovingly how bonnie you were. Your child's mind would store this information, and a self-image of yourself as cuddly and loveable would be stored in your thoughts. As an adult you still have an image of yourself as cuddly which you find hard to let go. Let go you must. You need a new self-image; that of a successful slimmer.

## THINK SLIM STRATEGIES
• Make Think Slim Self-Image/Self-Esteem Cards:

> I used to be a Dieting Disaster
> Now I'm a Successful Slimmer

• Amend your own words to suit your situation.

# ASSIST YOURSELF!
## Identify your
## Negative Wizards

Carrie had lost 5 pounds/2 kilos in her first week of slimming. She was delighted but her delight was spoiled by the doubt she expressed in a wistful voice: 'I always start off so well, but then it all seems to go wrong . . . I don't know why . . .'

A very big reason why 'it all seems to go wrong' is that we are beset by influences – that I call 'Negative Wizards'. Negative Wizards are the powerful influences in our lives that are the saboteurs of our slimming. These saboteurs can be found in different aspects of our lives: in our life, in the shape of other people whom we know; all around us in our culture, in the messages given in advertisements on television, in books and magazines; and in ourselves – that is, in our automatic thoughts and our habits.

To slim successfully, first you need to identify the Negative Wizards that have been sabotaging your efforts to become and stay slim. Each slimmer is unique, with a different lifestyle (eg, mum-at-home, working woman, business man, manual worker, retired person, teenage girl, student, and so on), and therefore has different Negative Wizards influencing her or him. However, from the list of Negative Wizards that are presented here, you will soon recognise which ones sabotage your efforts to slim. Forewarned is forearmed, and this chapter will also give you ideas about how to avoid the sabotage. Your slimming success will be much more likely when you have ways of shooting down your saboteurs.

Gina, a hairdresser whose hair was in better condition than her body, identified her two fatal Negative Wizards in the first fortnight of attending my group. They were both within herself, and they were her 'That Li'l Bit thinker' and 'Nega-thinker' selves.

'That Li'l Bit won't hurt,' she'd think to herself, over and over again . . . as another Li'l Bit in her mouth put another Li'l Bit on her hips. If she wasn't eating just another little bit, she was 'Nega-thinking': thinking how miserable all this slimming effort was, and depressing herself into the sort of depression that can only be lifted by a currant bun or three.

But Gina conquered her unhelpful and negative thinking, and along with it, her excess weight problems. Gina remains slim, over one year later. Now her customers admire her figure as well as her hair.

Sometimes, slimmers are reluctant to be honest with this task of identifying their Negative Wizards.

Cathy was one who declared that she had *no* Negative Wizards. She loved chocolate but never ate any, her married life was perfect, her children were manageable, her eating habits impeccably healthy. She was defending her image, but the roundy-boundy shape of her 5-foot body belied her words. Why was she defending herself so? It is not so surprising. Most of us have been made to feel so guilty about our eating and our overweight, and have been insulted and scoffed at, that to prevent ourselves from withering away inside as a person, we defend ourselves by denying both our guilt and our responsibility.

Now, there's no blame. This time, it's different. I shall not be damning you for your eating 'dreadfulness'. Anything 'awful' that you've done, I've probably done! Or, even if I've not done it, I've heard it all before. Nor is it helpful for *you* to chastise yourself with silent words such as: 'I ought to be ashamed of myself! I'm hopeless! I'm a Dieting disaster – a fat slob!'

The aims of this chapter are:

1 To help you to *identify* your Negative Wizards. As you identify the saboteurs of your previous slimming efforts, you will avoid blaming yourself; you will think something like: 'Oh yes, that's me – that's interesting!'
2 To help you to eliminate their destructive power. You will aim to replace them with more helpful influences. Worry not, for you will also be shown strategies to help you replace your Negative Wizards with your own Positive Proddings.

So, hunt those Negative Wizards.

## 1 NEGATIVE WIZARDS IN YOUR LIFE

You may recognise that people in your life behave as Negative Wizards; at home, at work, in your family, in your social circle.

### THE COMMANDER

You are tucking in, moderately, to the favourite chocolate that you have chosen as part of your slimming strategy.

The Commander (your spouse, friend, mother, bus driver, petrol attendant, passer-by) spots you and accuses loudly (for all to hear): 'You shouldn't be eating that! You'll get fat!' (The Commander is full of 'Shouldn't-bes': you shouldn't be eating this, or doing that.)

Automatically, guilt stabs at you, even though it's unnecessary, for your chocolate was the 'little bit of what you fancy' that's very necessary to a civilised slimmer. Guilt, conditioned into place by years of diet-think, mugs your mind and your calm control is shattered. Another binge is threatening.

Something similar used to happen to me every Friday, when I collected my 'reward' chocolate Little Egg, from my village shop. The female mass of 16 stones/100 kilos in a pinafore, overflowing behind the counter, never failed to make some Commander remark on the theme of 'Shouldn't be'. I could have replied cuttingly, but then I was losing weight, and she was still miserably massive. There's enough unkindness in this world. You can have a Think Slim answer that's effective but not unkind: 'I'm losing weight *and* eating some chocolate. Suits me.'

Another very common Commander remark (usually word-for-word!) is: 'You shouldn't be eating that. You're supposed to be on a diet!' Your Think Slim answer is more useful if it is learned, ready to trip off your tongue: 'I'm *not* on a diet. I'm slimming, and I *can* have this.' By 'slimming', I mean losing excess weight gradually, in a civilised way, adopting new ways of nutritious and delicious eating that will last for a lifetime after that fat is lost.

Alternatively, you might find that The Commander is in your own head; you, chastising yourself as you chew, an influence from years of Diet Think: 'I shouldn't be eating . . .' If so, repeat your Think Slim answer to yourself: 'I'm not on a diet. I'm slimming and I can have this.' Repeat it often, often, often.

## COUNTERACT WITH THINK SLIM

- Be prepared for negative encounters of The Commander kind, and ready with your answer. To answer is better than to ignore, for answering asserts your own self and your right to choose how to slim; answering empowers you, and adds to your overall confidence; saying aloud the Think Slim words that you believe in, fixes them even more firmly in your thoughts, and maximises your chances of slim success.

  The answer is better if it reinforces your Think Slim approach, refuses to allow inappropriate guilt, and avoids shattering your slimming composure.

- Learn your answer, the Think Slim phrase: 'I'm *not* on a diet, I'm slimming, and I *can* have this.'

- If The Commander persists, don't be drawn into an argument. Repeat your Think Slim answer, *in exactly the same words*, as often as it's necessary.

## THE JAILER

Sometimes, slimmers ask someone near and dear to them to be their Jailer. Sara asked her husband to lock the kitchen cupboard where the biscuits and cakes were kept, to prevent her from sneaky-snacking.

It may seem like a good idea, but it is not, for it is abdicating your own responsibility and acting like a naughty child who can't be trusted.

It's dangerous because it feeds your own 'I'm useless' self-image. A person who believes he or she is useless will *be* useless.

Women in particular are prone to play the 'Useless-little-me' game, because they have been conditioned to believe it is a 'feminine' way to behave and that it pleases men. It does please some men, but it's not worth the price, for by playing little girl you sabotage your slimming efforts. Then, anyway, you run the risk of not pleasing him because you're overweight!

Janine was an 'I'm-so-useless' eyelash fluttering man-pleaser, wearing a Kylie bow in her hair and alternating her clothes style between Laura Ashley Romantic and vamp. Her weight blossomed as sweets slunk out of her pocket and into her mouth all day long as she worked, in an attempt to calm her anxiety about winning this man, or changing that one. She only lost weight when the latest man was into healthy eating, became her Jailer, and trailed her on long unaccustomed walks. But, the more reluctance he showed about leaving his wife, the more weight she gained.

Janine is convinced that she's unlucky with men and with her weight. So, her story has no happy ending (well, not yet; there's hope for everyone). Until she is prepared to recognise and change the game she's playing, she will continue to be unfortunate with both men and her figure. Luck plays no part. We choose our weight just as we choose our men.

Playing the game of 'Useless-little-me – please help me and be my Jailer' undermines your efforts to become a self-empowered slimmer, making your own rational decisions and choices, and taking responsibility for your own actions.

Furthermore, having a Jailer hardly ever works in the long term. For, it is likely that you will, like an adolescent, rebel against this authority (yes, despite the fact that you asked for it; there's 'nowt so funny as folk'). Then you will get yourself some of that forbidden fruit (well, biscuits) by hook or by crook, and feel good about your secret victory over the Jailer. Unfortunately, it is no victory; for it is you, with your chosen target of slimness, who has defeated yourself.

Also, if you have a row with the Jailer (or harbour a resentment) you may eat to 'get back' at him/her – but you are the (fatter) loser!

All of this is not to suggest that you try to do without support. Support is necessary and good, but you need to ask for what support you need, clearly, without playing games. Asking for a Jailer is not asking for support, it is a way of becoming dependent, then rebellious, and staying overweight.


## COUNTERACT WITH THINK SLIM

- Don't ask (or allow) anyone to take the role of your personal Jailer. Take responsibility for yourself.
- Think Slim: 'I am My Own Keeper.'

## THE PUT-DOWNER:

'You're *not* on another diet!' 'What scheme is it *this* time? Magic Marmalade? Tomato and Treacle?'

The Put-downer jokes, but it's no joke to you. Or, The Put-downer is downright insulting: 'You know you'll never do any good!' 'I'm fed up with your greediness!'

The effect of The Put-downer's words is to sap your confidence, lower your self-esteem, and undermine your self-image which you are trying to build as an effective slimmer.

The words prompt your own doubts. Perhaps you won't do any good, and you have been on rather a lot of diets before, and you're still overweight . . . and maybe it is silly trying again, and well, yes, you do seem greedy sometimes (but he eats more than you!) . . . and oh well! it's probably not worth the effort. You might as well have a Mars Bar!

If you allow free rein to such negative thoughts, you are dooming yourself to failure with your slimming. Such negative thoughts are in your head, and you are able to change them.

So argue back, first aloud to The Put-downer, and also silently and repeatedly to the negative side of yourself that The Put-downer has encouraged.

Replace the negative image of yourself with a more positive 'can-do' image.

### COUNTERACT WITH THINK SLIM

- Your Think-Slim Answers:
  'I'm *not* on a diet. I'm slimming and I'm doing fine.'
    'This time it's a civilised scheme of eating!'
    'This time I'm doing fine.'
    'I'm not greedy. I used to eat too much sometimes, but I don't do it now and I'm not greedy.'
- Refuse to be drawn into an argument with the Put-downer; she/he won't be convinced, and your confidence may be undermined. Simply repeat your Think Slim phrases, above, as often as is necessary.
- If you feel your confidence slipping, repeat to yourself, many times: 'I'm slimming and I'm doing fine.'
- Put-downers often repeat the same 'insult'. *Notice* those used on you. *Prepare* your answer, learn it, and repeat it to him/her, as often as it takes . . .
- If the Put-downer is your spouse, and he/she is sabotaging your confidence, a controlled chat is needed. Choose a quiet and suitable time to say you want a chat. (Don't begin when he/she has just settled down to watch hishe/her favourite television programme.) Without losing your temper, explain that you know he/she has your best interests at heart, but tell how hishe/her comments are undermining you; say what would be helpful to you. Show this book to The Put-downer, and together discuss this approach to slimming. Perhaps your spouse might want to lose a bit of excess weight too?

## THE SPOILER

Between them, Sue's friends bought her fifteen boxes of chocolates as Christmas gifts. With friends like these, what slimmer needs enemies?

Why do they do this? Perhaps they just don't give the matter too much thought; buying chocs is an easy way to get through gift shopping. Or, perhaps it's habit. They have always bought you chocs, and let's face it, you've not shown any real reluctance about it before.

Or, maybe they are trying to sabotage your slimming. They see you, at last succeeding at becoming slimmer. This is not the good old Big Brenda that they are comfortable with. They would feel more comfortable with you the way you were. Or, maybe they are a little green-eyed at your success, for perhaps they would like to lose some weight. So, maybe not even consciously, they apply a little sabotage. It may not be presents; it may be a casual offering: 'Go on, spoil yourself!' tempts The Spoiler, waving the high-calorie goodies under your all-too-willing nose.

But it will spoil you. It will spoil your efforts, your figure, your fitness and your health. Spoiling yourself with high-cal treats is another saboteur.

'This little bit won't hurt you!' they encourage. OK, you know that 'a little' won't hurt you, if it really is a little and you haven't had 'a little' seventeen times already today. You must decide – honestly – whether your day has calorie-space for 'a little'. And whether you can restrict yourself to a little! Margie always gives us the timely reminder that biscuits are made on elastic. Eat one, and the invisible elastic whisks the rest into your mouth without a by-your-leave!

Joanna created the best Think Slim answer to this Negative Wizard: 'No, it won't hurt me – because I'm not having it.' If you don't wish to be so definite as Joanna (who lost over 2 stones/13 kilos three years ago and is still slim), then ask yourself this question:

'Do I really want it? Yes I do.

But I'll allow for it; I promise to!'

OR

'Do I really want it? No I don't!

Shall I eat it? No I won't!'

When you are making the decision whether or not you really want some foodie-treat, always ask yourself: 'Is it worth its calories?' Everything you eat has a cost, just as do items like clothes, cars or furniture that you buy. Just as you decide whether goods are worth their cash/credit price, you need to decide whether food is worth its calorie price. Remember that your aim is to be slim. Now, is this food worth its calories?

When Cathy weighed in at a weekly Think Slim meeting she'd had her best weight loss ever. She explained how she'd achieved it. 'I asked myself all week: is it worth its calories? And most of the time, it wasn't!'

However, maybe your answer sometimes is: 'yes, I want it and it is worth the calories.'

'Yes, but I say I'll make up for things, and then I don't,' confessed Amy, with a sigh. If you are like Amy, then there are three options open to you.
1  Stay overweight.
2  Recognise that you can't trust yourself, and always say no! Julia, admirably succeeding at slimming despite a health battle for her young child who has a brain tumour, swore that making a card with the 'No I don't' rhyme written on it and carrying it around in her purse was the key to her success.
3  Change yourself. Keep promises you make to yourself. If you made a promise to someone else (such as 'I'll meet you at the cinema at 8 pm'), you would do that, wouldn't you? (If your answer is 'no' – you need to give yourself lessons in being an acceptable person, now.)
Treat yourself with the same respect that you treat others. Whatever you promise to yourself, do it. Don't ask yourself, 'shall I?' Just do it. Repeat to yourself: 'I always do what I say.' Repeat the words often enough, put it into practice often, and you will have changed yourself for the better, for a lifetime. Then, you will find that you get what you want out of life much more often.

## COUNTERACT WITH THINK SLIM
- Make Think Slim cards, with the 'Do I really Want It?' rhymes written one on each side of the card(s). Learn the words. Carry them around with you. Use the questions when faced with Spoiler treats.
- Also, always ask yourself: 'Is It worth its Calories?'
- Your Positive Think Slim answer to 'Go on, spoil yourself!': 'No thanks, spoil myself is exactly what I *don't* want to do.'

## THE SMOTHERER
The Smotherer claims to be looking after you. The Smotherer is often a mother, but may be a spouse or a friend.
'You shouldn't be slimming, with all those children to look after! You need your food with your job!' is the repeated smothering advice that Daisy, who is a child minder, receives from her anxious mother.
The Smotherer may have good intentions, but we know that the road of slimming sabotage can be paved with other people's good intentions.
'You need sugar for energy,' spouts father-in-law Joe, in ignorance, while imperiously spooning sugar into my coffee. If something similar happens to you, do as I do: smile sweetly and say that you're sweet and energetic enough, thank you, and refuse the offending drink. You may not be able to teach the old dog new tricks, particularly when he doesn't want to learn, so don't try giving him the facts on sugar. (If you don't know the facts on sugar, you can find them in the Nutrition Matters section, page 169). However, do always refuse to consume the offending drink, for to give in will simply encourage other attempts at bossily sabotaging you. This approach also applies to any high calorie food that others press on you, under the guise of doing you good or treating you.

**COUNTERACT WITH THINK SLIM:**
- Think Slim answer: 'No, thanks. I'm slimming and getting fitter and healthier!'
- An alternative answer is that 'It doesn't suit my stomach, thank you'. The Smotherer will assume your tummy is delicate (while you and I know it's overweight), and is more likely to accept your refusal.
- Remind yourself that you are in charge of your life: you don't need a Smotherer.

# 2 NEGATIVE WIZARDS IN OUR CULTURE

'That's me!' 'That's just the way I am!' Those are both phrases that we often hear. But just how did we get to be 'the way we are'?

Most of us like to think that we were born the way we are: unique – 'me'. However, from psychology studies, we know that that is just not so. From almost the moment of birth we begin to 'learn', to become who we are. We 'learn' from the many people and influences around us.

Influences from our culture play their part. Every day of our lives we receive 'messages' from television, advertisements, magazines, pop songs, and so on. We learn that the best shape for women is thin; that Real Men drink lager; that mums cook and dads earn money; that cream cakes are naughty but nice.

These and many other messages are all around us, and often we take hardly any conscious notice. Yet the messages are noticed by our brain. Perhaps you can recognise how easily you learn the tune or words of a pop song and find yourself humming along, without having sat down and made any deliberate effort to learn it.

Similarly, we take in all sorts of messages (many about eating and slimming), and unless we make ourselves aware and challenge the messages, they are stored in our brain-computer, to insidiously influence our thinking for the rest of our life. Companies spend vast sums on their advertisements because they know that people *are* influenced by them.

'Subliminal' advertising – where a message is flashed so fast on screen that the eye does not see it but it is registered in the brain – is, rightly, illegal in this country. For its messages influence people without them even being consciously aware that a message exists. It has dangerous, brain-washing potential in unscrupulous hands. Yet you will see subliminal videos and audio cassettes offered for sale some of which claim to help you to slim. You listen or watch such products whilst having no conscious idea what the messages are. I cannot recommend them because I believe that we should have none of what we cannot check, think about, and challenge.

Unfortunately, many cultural influences are in fact more Negative Wizards, which have helped to spoil our slimming previously and could undermine our Think Slim approach, unless we become aware of them and counteract them. On the following pages, you will find some of the Cultural Negative Wizards for you to chase out of your life.

## EAT, DRINK AND BE MERRY!

'Make Your Journey Worthwhile.' Where was it, do you suppose, that I spotted this advertising slogan? A travel agent? Inter-city train? No, it was on a machine dispensing chocolate bars.

In our materialistic culture, consumption is encouraged – including the consumption of food. Especially consumption of high-calorie treats which we are brainwashed to believe are essential to our pleasure. The misleading message is that to enjoy yourself, eating is essential! 'A Visit to McDonalds Makes Your Day!' sings out the television advertisement. Once, if we went to the cinema we were offered merely an ice-cream, but now there's a wide miscellany of munchie business, and popcorn comes not in packets but in bucketfuls. 'Nice, though,' I can hear you mutter. Of course it is. Except that it has side effects. It makes us fat. Remind yourself of what you really want – to be slim and fit to enjoy your life.

'I feel just like going to the cinema!' Julie informed her husband one evening. But he knew her very well. He eyed her suspiciously.

'No, you don't,' he diagnosed. 'You just want an ice-cream!'

'And he was right!' she admitted, with a giggle, recognising that she had been kidding herself. (So they didn't go, she didn't bother with ice-cream, and she did reach her target weight, which she still keeps, three years later.)

At one of my local cinemas, the woman who is wedged behind the munchies counter is a splendid advert for her wares; at least 16 stones/100 kilos of flab is straining at her uniform. So, I keep my eyes on her, not her sweetie bags, and I think to myself: 'and that's the price I'd pay for all that munchie business!' Then I'm content to glide past with nothing more than my ticket in my hand.

### COUNTERACT WITH THINK SLIM

- Notice the cultural dictates to eat; scoff at them (rather than at the food they're pushing); create Think Slim answers to counteract the messages.
- Repeat the Think Slim slogan when you see an overweight example of those who accept the cultural instructions eat, eat, eat: 'and that's the price *I'd* pay for all that munchie business!'

## INSTANTISM

Instant coffee. Three Minute Microwave Ready-meal.

Thin Thighs in 10 Days.

*Flatten Your Stomach in 15 Days*: a recent book-title.

'Lose seven pounds in seven days,' exhorts a newspaper doctor.

Herbal slim-tablets, Bai Lin Tea, Grapefruit Pills: all 'easy' potions – without dieting.

Learn to speak French in no time. Play the keyboard in a day.

Cultural messages promise instantism, and condition us to expect it.

Would you buy a book that was entitled *A Flat Stomach in Three Years*? Yet it may be a more realistic theme for those who are heavily overweight.

When we begin to diet, by when do we want to be slim? Tomorrow morning. Or yesterday. Certainly no later than three weeks. Research indicates that just over 50 per cent of dieters give up before one month.

'I've tried every diet,' sighed Mary, still overflowing with flesh. 'None of them worked.' The truth is that Mary only 'tried' every diet; never followed them, consistently, for a long period of time.

'But that's hard!' she protests, at the very idea. Yes, it is hard. But it's also real life, not the Instantism of advertisements.

We need to challenge the idea that the Instantism that is OK for coffee (yet even not so nice as the slowly perked Real Thing) *cannot* be possible for slimming.

## COUNTERACT WITH THINK SLIM

- Think Slim recognises realism, and corrects the faulty thinking that sighs for Slimming Instantism.
- Set realistic short-term targets, and also long-term ones. 'In one year's time I shall be . . .' (read the section later called Target Yourself, page 127). If the very idea of long-term targets strikes horror into your Instantism-conditioned mind, you need to work on this issue, or you will doom yourself to failure and fatness (or the fat-thin yo-yo, forever).
- Think of a daffodil bulb. Fat and round with lots of layers. (Remind you of anyone?) It is planted in September, and has to work all autumn right through to the spring, before it emerges in all its glory – slim, elegant, bright and nodding its triumphant head to the world. Think of yourself as rather like a daffodil bulb. Work for as long as it takes to become slim.
- When you see an advert which is clearly nonsense, remind yourself that it's rubbish. 'What do you think of this one?' I call to my slimmers, waving yet another Miracle-Slim ad in my hand.

    'Rubbish!' they yell in laughing response, their purses remaining firmly shut.

Send a letter of complaint to the Advertising Standards Authority, so that the ad must be withdrawn. Don't get tempted to part with your money. Get angry that people are trying to con you out of your money again. If you remain tempted when you see yet another such advert, recognise this as a sign that your mind is still gripped by Instantism. Scotch your 'Is it worth a try?' thoughts, repeatedly, with those of 'Rubbish! Rubbish!'

## NEVER TOO THIN

'I'd love to be a stone thinner – but I don't know if I can stand another diet!' Sara declared dramatically, tossing her elegantly tousled fair hair, her bold jewellery jangling in chorus. I surveyed her five feet eight inch (1·7 metre) frame and her short sharp jacket with its very short sharp skirt. She looked wonderful, yet dissatisfaction was pulling at her lips.

It was Wallis Simpson, the Duchess of Windsor, who reputedly pronounced that a woman could never be too thin or too rich. She was thin, thin, thin (stick-insect extraordinaire), but I doubt it was her thinness that caused the heir to the throne to abdicate rather than forget her. She was not only too thin, she was wrong.

Why *should* women look like Adrian Mole aged 13¾? It's OK for Adrian Mole, but even he will grow out of it. For the rest of us, let's look like women, because that is who we are. When Mother Nature was dishing out the jobs in that Great Job Centre in the Sky, she decided, for better or worse, that women were to be the portion of the human species that gave birth. Her design consultants insisted that frontal lumps for feeding the young were a cost-effective idea, and that women should also have a natural talent for laying down fat, especially on the hips, tum and thighs, probably so that come the famine, they stood a better chance of survival and thereby give a better chance to the offspring. ('Survival of the species' was, of course, the idea, rather than 'fulfilment of women'.)

Perhaps nobody told Wallis Simpson. It is reputed that she spent her life rationing herself to one skimpy meal per day. For most of us, that's an undesirable price for thinness.

It is, of course, not only the influence of Wallis Simpson, whose name may well be totally unknown to many of the current generation of slimmers. More recently, there has been another influential First Lady in the form of teeny-weeny scraggy Nancy Reagan, setting a standard of thinness that's unnatural and unattainable by healthy and happy means. In Britain, the standard of over-lean and lanky is set by Princess Diana, another superfluous dedicated follower of pin-thin perfectionism.

Then there is also the women's fashion industry, parading its wares on lollipop sticks called models, and enticing us by example to superhuman slimming efforts or damning us to a sense of total inadequacy (even if we're a size 12).

Magazines splash fashion pages with photographed emaciations displaying, along with the clothes they wear, that Very Thin is In. Editors are heard trying to defend their indefensible position with mutterings about it's Not Their Fault – it's the only size they can get from the Fashion Houses – while the Fashion Houses do not deign to disturb themselves from their arrogant, silent, ivory, Thin towers.

Even the plastic mannequins that stand in shop windows have been redesigned over the years into thinner versions of their former selves. Even a man-made Marilyn Monroe would appear overweight in today's climate.

The thin conditioning process starts very early. Young girls play with Barbie and Cindy dolls that are no more than little plastic poles in hi-fashion clothes.

A 15-year-old girl demonstrates, in a letter to a national newspaper, the pressure upon teenage life to be thin. She is 'fed up' with 'the supposedly perfect bodies that the media keeps throwing at us'.

She continues: 'I cannot eat a square meal without feeling a surge of guilt, and three of my girl friends are anorexic. None of my girlfriends eat breakfast, half skip lunch, and some go for days without eating anything because they are so desperate for that "perfect" body.' (*Daily Express*, 2 October, 1991.)

Even some mature adult women stare miserably into a full length mirror, and, although faced with a fine slim body, see only lumps and hated fat. Paula stood on the scales in front of me and wrinkled her nose in disgust at her weight; she had reached the weight target that we had set together, but she wanted to be thinner. She poked furiously at her hips. 'Look, look at all this fat,' she groaned.

'Do you know what it is?' I began, gently. 'It's your hips. They are there because you're a woman . . .'

'It's not fair!' protested Amy passionately. Amy is slenderly slim with a petite bone structure, fine skin and spectacular naturally blonde hair that cascades way down her elegant spine. Always careful about her eating, she has always been slim. However, she continues to protest: 'I've been dieting for about six weeks and I've been living on nothing but water melon for ages, and I'm still not as thin as the magazine models!'

'It's not fair,' I began to respond, 'that you are being so cruel to your own body, and it's not fair that women's magazines prompt you to be so thin!'

We wrangled; she protested: 'Well, they do look beautiful.'

Beautiful? Beauty is in the eye of the beholder, and unfortunately we beholders have been increasingly conditioned into worshipping the unworthy: Lowry-like legs and hollow stomachs that are silently screaming for nourishment. As beauty, we are being sold the Empress's New Clothes.

It's not fair. Remember bound feet? The awful power that a culture can wield over its beauty-beholders is illustrated by Chinese women's bound feet, where mutilation became a sign of beauty and sexual attractiveness. Unenlightened Mothers enthused about crippling the feet of their poor daughters; puppet-daughters willingly bore the agonies and shuffled 'daintily' and 'femininely' along on their crippled toes. Eastern men – conditioned as equally as their womenfolk – drooled over this 'beauty', just as their conditioned Western counterparts might lust over thin thighs.

'It certainly is not fair,' I repeated to Amy. 'When you see skinny models with Lowry-like legs, think of bound feet. Don't let your mind be bound by the conditioning of the Think Thinners.'

Such realistic Think Slim convinced Amy. 'I think I'll go out for a meal tonight,' she mused.

'Chinese restaurant?' I joked. Now, Amy is wisely slim; and we still often mention 'bound feet'.

Some women become totally obsessed with the fat image that they think they see, and lose their sense of proportion. They acquire a distorted body-image, and their thoughts prompt them to believe they are still fat, even while they are wasting away, anorexically, into ill-health and even to death. Dying to be thin . . . literally.

Other women are so desperate to fulfil the injunction to be thin that they allow themselves to eat but then purge their body with laxatives or force themselves to be sick, to get rid of the calories. At first, it can seem to some women as if they are having the best of both worlds, having your cake and eating it too, while attaining that elusive thinness. They see their body as something separate from themselves, to be purged and punished and maltreated to make it conform to impossible demands. It is both sad and dangerous. Sad that they feel so compelled to perform, marionette-like, to the destructive tune of others; dangerous that they inflict such unnatural and damaging practices on their body, for, over a period of time, the poor beleaguered body degenerates.

Men do not suffer from these extreme conditioning demands upon their psyche and their body. However, men are conditioned too – to expect thinness in their women. Well, not quite thinness. For, the cultural fantasy woman that our men are brainwashed to want has a Page Three top, tiny hips, a non-existent tum and skinny legs six feet long – but yet is not as tall as they are; in other words, an impossible freak. They compare the female in their life with the livin' doll they drool after, and the real woman is found wanting . . . and she knows it. Knows it with angst and anxiety and guilt and a new diet.

So, fashion and culture combine to create the destructive 'oughta-bee' syndrome: you 'ought-to-be' thin . . . thin . . . thinner. Not thin enough equals not good enough, shouts our culture. Never thin enough. Get into a size 6 and they'll demand you slide down to a size 4. How long before the first size 'Minus 2' is in the shops?

It's not good enough that women be subjected to such unnatural nonsense. Nor is it good enough that we allow ourselves to accept it.

Now this is not to agree with the Fat Liberation Movement, which preaches that Fat is OK; even beautiful. Fat does not liberate us. It makes us clumsy, sweaty, tired, awkward, strained, unfit, even ill. Less able to conceive a child, less able to bloom throughout pregnancy, less able to romp and run with toddlers. One famous fat lady is reported as saying candidly: 'I'm fat so I sweat a lot.' Is that a liberated, enjoyable way to live?

Fat as beautiful? We could believe anything if we're brainwashed. However, Mother Nature is unlikely to have intended the human species to think of fat as beautiful, because being fat is so patently unhelpful for the survival of the cave-people she created.

So, both men and women need to refuse to allow cultural influences to trap them into the extremes of either 'Thin' or 'Fat'. Moderation is the wise way, a combination of healthy and happy. Slim is the aim, because Slim Living is More Enjoyable Living.

## COUNTERACT WITH THINK SLIM

- Slim Think: women should look like women – not like stick-insects or Adrian Mole, aged 13¾.
- Wear your womanly lumps with pride! (but don't kid yourself that your excess fat is a womanly lump!). Hips and thighs are OK in realistic womanly proportions.
- Think Slim: thin is unhealthy and unnecessary. Slim Living is More Enjoyable Living.
- Look at those fashion models in criticism, *not* admiration.
- Speak your criticisms aloud – and set other women free.

## *OUGHTA-BEE . . . PERFICK*

She oughta-bee: Ms Perfick Body, the Perfick Cook, Mrs Perfick Mum, the Perfick Boardroom Highflyer, the Absolutely Perfick Fragrant Wife, the Perfick Bedroom Sex Kitten, the Never-a-Slip-Up Slimmer.

He oughta-bee: The Perfick Chairman of The Board, the Perfick Breadwinner, the Perfick Father, the Perfick Brave Chap, the Perfick Lover, the Perfick New Man, the Perfick Gentleman, the Perfick Bit o' Rough; the Wonderful Weight Loser.

Advertisements exhort us to Perfick-tionism. So do pop songs such as the recent hit 'It's Got to Be . . . Perfect'.

The One Commandment: You oughta-bee Perfick. Don't accept anything less.

'I'm a perfectionist,' you hear others say, with pride. That makes them feel superior, and puts you in your place. Don't be tempted to join them. The Perfectionists have a problem. Probably it stems from an upbringing where they have had to be best before they could feel accepted and loved. At worst, Perfectionists are doomed to an anxious rat-race of a life, because they can never be sure that they are perfick enough.

So, many of them can be found signing ill-afforded cheques in Harley Street for nose-jobs, breasts perked with silicone and lips pouted with collagen, thighs reduced, fat sucked out, a nip here and a few tucks there. Once it all seemed the province of the over-wealthy under-active ageing American, but increasingly women as young as in their twenties feel not perfick enough, and even in conservative Britain in 1990 some ten thousand perfick-seekers bared their breasts to the cosmetic enlarger.

A whole technological rebuild can cost £20,000 in Britain and the pain is thought, by obsessives, to be cheap at the price. Some return repeatedly, addicted to the pursuit of perfick-tionism. It is common enough for psychiatrists to label the addiction – dysmorphophobia.

With so many cultural dictates descending upon us to be perfick, we must be strong to avoid the temptation to join in. I have an excellent piece of advice: 'If you feel the urge to be Perfick coming on, go and lie down till you've kicked it away.'

Notice the 'oughta-bee Perficks'. Laugh at them. Refuse to accept 'oughta-bees'. You can be what *you* want to be. If others don't like it that's their problem. This is not to say that you do not consider the feelings of others. This is not to take a 'let it all hang out' and 'I'm telling you the brutal truth, mate . . .' approach, reminiscent of some of the psycho-babble cultures of the Sixties.

Other people can be part of your equation. That is, the equation you use to choose how to live your life. You consider them, and their feelings, but they have no right to tell you what you oughta-bee. Especially when they tell you that you oughta-bee Ms/Mr Perfick Slimmer.

Moyra didn't arrive at the group one night. She phoned me to explain that her husband said she shouldn't come anymore because she oughta-bee getting better results; she wasn't losing weight quickly enough.

'Quickly enough for whom?' I asked. Whose body is it, anyway? Be your own un-perfick person.

## COUNTERACT WITH THINK SLIM
- Banish 'oughta-bees' from your thoughts. You can be what *you* want to be. If others don't like it, that's their problem.
- If any urge to be perfick hits you, go and lie down till you've kicked it away.
- Replace oughta-bees with wanna-bees, plus will-bees.
- *You* decide your own wanna-bees and will-bees. Talk them over with understanding friends, or a professional counsellor.
- Write them down; read them often; plan your action towards them; review your progress and amend your action as necessary.
- Think Slim: I am my own un-perfick person.

## THE SUPER-SLIMMER SYNDROME
This takes two forms:
1 There is the competition between slimmers as to who can lose weight quickest, and so walk away from the scales wearing that 'Aren't I just the Super-slimmer' smug smile.

Some slimming clubs encourage this, and every four weeks declare one of their members as 'Slimmer of the Month'. Maybe it seems like a good idea. It isn't.

Once, I could have won a Slimmer of the Month title. That was when I lost twelve pounds in twelve days. I was ecstatic about myself and the diet. (Did your Super-slimmer-conditioned ears prick up? Are your thoughts already shouting out, 'How? How? Tell me how!'? Tut, tut!) Well, it's not quite true that I was ecstatic. I actually felt almost suicidal. I just wanted to curl up my (beautifully slim) body into a quiet corner and resign from the human race.

I went to my doctor, thinking I must have caught some new disease. I had – the Super-slimmer Syndrome. I had starved my body and my brain of food and nourishment, of vitamins and minerals; I had exercised wildly; and my poor beleaguered body and mind couldn't cope. Fortunately, I had a doctor who talked to me instead of reaching for his prescription pad. A new principle was fixed firmly in my thoughts. It is no use being slim if you are not fit. My slim-fit principle was born. Slim enough and Fit enough to enjoy life.

## COUNTERACT WITH THINK SLIM
- Refuse to compete with others to see who can lose weight quickest. Think, and say: 'It's taking as long as it needs.'
- Don't ask people: 'How quick did you lose . . .?' Instead, ask: 'How healthy and enjoyable was your eating?'
- Object to 'Slimmer of the Month' type competitions. *Every* slimmer is the Slimmer of the Month!
- Accept, gracefully, small weight losses. Think, and say, 'I'm on the Right Track!' Grow slim gracefully.

2 The second form of Super-slimmer Syndrome can be recognised by words such as: '13 Stones Lost!' (A scream from a recent advert – 13 stones equals 82½ kilos.) Well, yes, it's worth boasting about. But there are so many of these massive weight losses assaulting our ears that our hard-won loss of 1½ stones/9½ kilos hardly seems worth mentioning. So, instead of feeling delighted with our achievement, we see it as mundane, and deprive ourselves of a much-needed boost to our self-esteem. Every successful slimmer, whether they have lost 7 lbs/3 kilos or 17 stones/108 kilos, has achieved splendidly.

## COUNTERACT WITH THINK SLIM
- Think Slim: *Any* amount of weight lost is an achievement.
  I've lost it, I've done well, and I'm proud of it.
  I am my own Slimmer of the Month.

## *EXCESS-ISM*
'More' pleaded Oliver, with his hungry begging bowl. Oliver needed more; he knew real hunger. But our culture preaches that more means better. The more food we eat, the better time we must be having. If our plates groan with food, and we groan with indigestion, we must be enjoying ourselves.

'I was so full I could hardly move!' is said boastfully, cheerfully, self-admiringly. Restaurants are often recommended on the basis of how much is served. Quantity rules.

'Have another little drink' is the pressure at parties, lunches, weddings and even funerals. If you are drinking alcohol, you must be having a great time. If you're imbibing enough alcohol to float a battleship, it indicates that you are having a whale of a time. We are so conditioned by the notion that successful socialising means alcohol that we never question it. If someone wants no alcohol, they are boring. To be boring is to be the 1990's Pariah.

This all goes beyond 'eat, drink and be merry'; it's 'the more you eat and drink the merrier you be'. 'Merry' is what we call people when in fact they are showing symptoms of alcohol poisoning.

When Mara came to my slimming group, she used to have a great time out with her friends every Saturday night; and she knew she did because she drank eleven lagers. Apart from the damage from some 1100 calories, there was the potential damage to her body.

'If you don't drink that much, they call you boring,' she explained. We talked about resisting pressure from others. Would she throw herself off a cliff if they threatened to call her boring otherwise? Whose life is it, anyway? Whose body? Whose fat?

For men, the pressure to float in alcohol can be even greater. A Real Man doesn't eat quiche but he does drink, and the more he drinks, and the quicker, the more of a Man he is.

The whole issue of excess-ism needs careful and rational thought. We are like Pavlov's dogs, responding to the social situation with too much alcohol and without any rational thought. I don't suggest that people have to ban alcohol, but use it reasonably. If the thought of restricting your alcohol to a moderate level bothers, angers or irritates you, perhaps you need to be asking yourself whether you are already becoming addicted.

Moderate levels of alcohol are considered by doctors to be for men 21 units each week; for women 14 units. (Sorry, no equality!)

## ALCOHOL UNITS

One unit of alcohol is equal to any *one* of the following:

One unit equals:
*Beer/lager*  ½ pint/285 ml ordinary strength.
*Spirits*  One English standard pub measure (⅙ gill/25 ml).
NB: Scotland uses ⅕ gill/28 ml,
Northern Ireland ¼ gill/35 ml.
*Sherry*  One English standard pub measure (⅓ gill/50 ml).
NB: A 'schooner' glass of sherry = 2 units.
*Wine*  One glass, 4 fluid oz/113 ml
(Measures in British pubs may vary.)
*Vermouth/*
*Aperitif*  One English standard pub measure (¼ gill/35 ml).
*Liqueur*  One English standard pub measure (⅙ gill/25 ml).

Some drinks contain more than one unit:
½ pint strong lager, beer or cider = 2 units
½ pint extra strong lager or beer = 2½ units
Cocktails vary; one cocktail may have 3 to 4 units.
NB: 75cl bottle of wine = 8 units.

Low-alcohol wines and beers vary as to how 'low' they are; this depends on the percentage of alcohol remaining. Compare the percentage remaining, as shown on the label, to the usual full strength alcohol figure of between 8–12 per cent of volume for wines and about 4 per cent for beers.

## COUNTERACT WITH THINK SLIM
- Challenge excess-ism.
- Think Slim:
    We don't have to eat and drink too much to have a good time.
    Food and Drink – Quality not Quantity.

# 3 NEGATIVE WIZARDS IN YOURSELF

Do you sometimes feel as if you are a Jekyll and Hyde, as though there is a good and bad side of you, fighting it out in your own mind? Indeed, there are opposing 'selves' within us; what we might call your Negative Self, and your Positive Self.

The Negative Wizard in yourself is your Negative Self, which shows itself in how you think. Negative thinking is destructive of your optimism and perseverance. It whispers that you'll never get slim, that it's not worth it, or that you're hopeless and useless at slimming. This negative thinking becomes a habit, like a tape recording playing over and over again in your mind, and repeatedly sabotages your slimming efforts.

'I know I'm my own worst enemy,' sighs Sue dejectedly. Sue need not feel dejected. At least she has completed a first step. She has recognised that she, by how she thinks, is playing a destructive part among her slimming efforts. Next, she (and you) need to pinpoint exactly what types of Negative Wizard thinking patterns are within. Then Think Slim strategies can be created to fight back and replace them.

I am inviting you to identify your destructive thinking patterns, but not so as to heap blame upon your head and tell yourself it's all your own fault. You need not inflict such mental torture on yourself, because it is not helpful. Only when you have identified your destructive thinking habits can you begin to replace them with those that will encourage slimming success.

So, read the following, ready to acknowledge some (all?) of these negative thinking patterns as yours.

## THE WOODEN LEG SYNDROME

'You can't expect me to slim, I've got a wooden leg . . .' For 'wooden leg', read a mother in hospital, a fractious baby, an unfaithful husband, the decorating to do, visitors staying, a sick parrot . . .

They are all excuses.

There will never be a 'perfect', totally stressless time, for you to slim. It is like the man in the play, *Waiting for Godot*. Godot never came, and the man who waited had wasted his life, waiting. The 'perfect time' for slimming will never come for you.

Why postpone your life? I often remind myself and my slimmers: This

Is Not a Dress Rehearsal. This (as far as we can know) is the only life that we have. Don't waste it. Slim now. So you can make the most of this life, now. Make efforts not excuses.

The best (worst?) excuse I ever heard was from a roly-poly woman who had not lost weight all week, and explained: 'I've been staying at my brother's all week and he's got gas central heating and I'm used to solid fuel.' The worst excuse I ever read was on the front of a certain Sunday tabloid newspaper that is not famous for its news: a picture of a scantily clad woman of immense proportions was accompanied by the caption: 'A dirty tattoo needle made me fat!'

The excuses just quoted are unusual in that they are so incredible but many people make excuses that sound plausible. The psychiatrist Freud termed it 'rationalising'. He suggested that we do this to 'defend' ourselves from attack by others. We also do it with ourselves – we 'kid' ourselves. It is almost as though the truth hurts too much, and we are unable to face our own guilt or responsibility. Besides, it's nice to eat, and if we rationalise, make our excuses, we can have our cake and eat it too – we eat without taking responsibility or feeling guilty. Unfortunately for us, although we can fool our mind, we can't fool our body. What we eat to excess turns to fat.

To be successful at slimming, to be self-empowered slimmers, we need to be brave enough to stop our rationalising. We can do that if we start being kinder and gentler with ourselves. If we throw away the guilt and the blame-game, we can be honest about why we are overweight.

There is one reason why we are overweight. We are overweight because we over-eat; that is, over-eat for our own unique body requirements and the amount of exercise we do. Think realistically to Think Slim: 'we are overweight because we over-eat'.

Whenever tempted to attribute excess weight to big bones or genetics, or to standing next to a bar of chocolate, or to the central heating, or simply 'I don't know why . . .', rethink realistically: 'we are overweight because we over-eat'. Stop making excuses and you can start to find solutions to why you are over-eating and find something more helpful to do instead.

## COUNTERACT WITH THINK SLIM
- Make a Think Slim Card:

> This Is Not A Dress Rehearsal.
> Life's Too Short To Live It Fat.
>
> Make Efforts not Excuses!

- Decide where to keep your card (or make more than one; use Post-it sticky notes and put them on your dressing table mirror; in your

kitchen; on your desk; by your bed; on a notice board).
- Re-read it often. Repeat it to yourself hundreds of times. Say it aloud. Discuss it with others.
- Repeat to yourself: 'We are overweight because we over-eat; no other reason.' Make a card stating it, if this is a particular issue for you.
- Identify your other personal 'excuses'. What other excuses do you make?

Write them here:                        Re-think them realistically, and
                                        write the truth:

......................................................................................

......................................................................................

......................................................................................

......................................................................................

......................................................................................

......................................................................................


## LIVING IN NEVER NEVER LAND

'I'll Never lose all this weight!'

'I'll Never get to my target weight!'

'I'll Never conquer this chocolate habit!'

'I'll Never get under 9 stones/57 kilos.'

'I've Never been under 10 stones/64 kilos in my life and I'll never get under!'

This is never-think that condemns us to 'Living in Never Never Land'. Every time we think to ourselves 'I'll never . . .' we make it more likely that we won't. For if we tell ourselves that we will never achieve something, we won't put all our efforts into trying. Because our efforts are half-hearted, slimming success is unlikely.

Additionally, we fail because our never-never thinking dooms us through the effect of what psychologists call the 'self-fulfilling prophecy'. This is the human tendency to perform only up to expectations. If you want to achieve great things, you must start with great expectations of yourself.

Even other people's low expectations can limit our performance if we listen to their views, doubt our own capabilities and reduce our efforts. This phenomenon has even been witnessed in school achievement and called the 'Pygmalion effect' after the story of how a 'common' flower girl was transformed into a lady through the expectations and teaching of Professor Higgins. To achieve your transformation into a permanently slim-fit person, you can use this book as your Professor Higgins, and stop yourself thinking your never-never thoughts.

If you think realistically, you know that it *is* possible to be slim; that the laws of nature insist that if you take in less calories than you use up, you will lose excess weight. My next comment may sound tough, but it reminds us of the truth and stops us kidding ourselves about our excess weight: when you slip into never-never thinking, remind yourself that there are no size 26s in starving Third World countries.

So, weight loss is possible through slimming; there are many examples of people having lost weight that has sat on them for decades. Joan is now down at a weight she has not enjoyed for over thirty years, before her children were born. But she's there now, and she's delighted to find she can slide her slimmer body into her son's TVR sports car. It's never too late, and you're never too old.

Betsy had lost over a stone to reach 11 stones 1 pound/70 kilos; she was pleased but slipping into never never land. 'I always get this far,' she began, 'but then I can't get any lower and I go back up again!' Certainly, if she sets a limit in her thoughts, she will set a limit to her achievement.

'You are subject to the same laws of nature as the rest of us,' I explain, 'and if you carry on slimming you will carry on losing weight to your sensible target. Do concentrate your thoughts and efforts this week and lose that bit to get you under this limit you have been setting yourself.'

Yes, Betsy did, and you can too.

However, there can be one 'never' that is a *helpful* thought, after you have reached your target weight: 'I'll *never* put all that weight back on!'

## COUNTERACT WITH THINK SLIM

- Every time you catch yourself thinking 'I'll never . . .', practise the 'Thought-stopping' Technique. Fiercely, think to yourself: 'STOP'.

    Then, consider this 'Never Never Land' you are condemning yourself to. Identify what it is you are thinking is 'never' possible. First, do check that the weight you want to be *is* realistic for your height, with a published chart or your doctor; then re-think your never never, positively. Replace it with: 'Of course I shall . . . ! All it takes is effort!'

    Repeat the words to yourself – and aloud to others – very often.

- If you, like Betsy, have your own 'psychological thought-block' about getting down to a weight you are near, concentrate all your thoughts and energies on attaining it. Ring a friend every day to state your determination aloud and to tell her/him about your eating and efforts. Do this daily until you have overcome your own induced weight-barrier.

## *NOT IN THE MOOD*

'I'm just not in the mood!' Anna announces, decisively. Not in the mood, that is, for slimming. She is ready to go away and lie down (eating and getting more overweight?) and wait for the right mood to arrive.

Moods, however, do not 'arrive' out of the blue. Our mood – how we feel – is determined by how we think.

Consider waking up one morning with the sun streaming through your bedroom window and you have one day off work to go for a picnic. What is your mood? Bright, enthusiastic, cheerful? What were your thoughts immediately you woke up? 'Oh, good, no work, picnic today, lovely sunny day – great, great, great!' Your positive thoughts have created your positive mood.

Now, imagine the same occasion, but instead of you waking to the sunshine, you see the summer sky pouring with rain and howling with wintry winds. Now, what are your first thoughts? 'Oh no! **** rain! I can't believe this! Now, what are we going to do about the picnic? My day off, ruined! Just my luck! Nothing goes right for me!' Now, what is your mood? Grumpy, disappointed, miserable.

The difference is in the weather (and you can't alter that), and in how you think about it (and you can alter that). Mr/Ms Holiday-maker could have avoided pinning all hopes on a picnic, not relying on the weather, and had some alternative and still attractive plans at the ready.

Similarly, if your mood is working against your slimming, remember that it is your thoughts that are causing your mood-problem.

'Isn't slimming miserable!' sighed Susie, expressing her recurrent thoughts.

'I don't think it's miserable,' responded Jennie. 'Slimming is doing something about my weight problem.'

Jennie's thoughts were positive, and so was her mood. Her weight loss was 5 stones/37½ kilos three years ago, and she remains slim.

As already explained, what you think affects what you feel. You can make your mood even worse with what psychologists call 'Catastrophising', which you and I know better as 'making a mountain out of a molehill'. It's like the roly-poly lady 'awfulising': 'Life must be *awful* if you can't eat everything you want!' Life isn't awful if you choose not to over-eat; life in the slim-fit lane is good, far better than in the fat. That woman was, when you looked at her huge bulk, literally making a mountain out of a molehill – out of herself.

## COUNTERACT WITH THINK SLIM

- Remember: we make and change our moods by the thoughts we choose to think. Misery thinking nurtures misery moods.
- If you're 'not in the mood' for slimming, *you* change your mood: read an inspiring success story in a slimming magazine; chat to a friend; play some cheerful and inspiring music ('I will survive' by Gloria Gaynor is a favourite of mine); brush your hair and experiment with some cosmetics; move yourself – activity often lifts a blue mood, so walk, run, dance (yes, all by yourself if necessary!), exercise, swim, use your bike. Don't 'wait' to 'feel like it' – do it! (Also see Step 3, on Motivation, page 117.)
- Refuse to make a mountain out of a molehill; refuse to join the 'Awfulising' game.

- Think Slim: 'It's not Slimming that's miserable – it's being over-weight.'

## THE OSTRICH POSITION

'I don't think I'll like it . . .' you muse doubtfully. 'It' is almost any suggestion for slimming that is new to you, maybe food or maybe exercise. The position is often accompanied by a wrinkled-up nose.

'Try some toasted bran in your slim-soup to make it more filling,' I suggest.

The wrinkled nose appears, and maybe a shudder: 'Ugh, I don't think I'll like it . . .'

'Don't bore yourself with the same old recipes,' I encourage. 'Try this . . .'

'What's in it? Ooooh, I don't think I'll like it . . .' Ms/Mr Ostrich responds.

Approaching slimming with an open mouth and a closed mind is not helpful.

It's the same with new interests as it is with food. Try swimming; or an exercise bike; or calligraphy; or sketching; or T'ai Chi. But Mr/Ms Ostrich isn't listening, for they already have their head in the sand. 'No, I don't think . . .' Don't Knock it till you've tried it! And don't try it while secretly absolutely determined to prove your doubts right and me wrong!

One slimmer who determined to try was Carron who, for her 35th birthday treat, went ice skating for the very first time, and loved it. I met an inspiring man who had discovered racing car Activity Days as his 89th birthday treat, and now, at 92 years bright, was on his third visit. (My husband and I were racing round too; thank goodness we haven't waited till our octogenarian years to try this fun.) The Ostriches miss out, just as do the 'Awfulising' fatties who wouldn't be able to squeeze their bodies into the slim racing-car shape. Another fine pleasure they're missing.

### COUNTERACT WITH THINK SLIM

- Cultivate an Open Mind. Don't knock it till you've tried it. Whenever someone suggests something new to you (whether it be food or a new interest or hobby), think, and say: 'Perhaps I'll like it. I'll have a try!'
- Make a Card. Draw an Ostrich with its head in the sand (no penalties if you can't draw!) and add, in big letters: NOT ME!

## 'I SHOULD BE SO LUCKY'

'Aren't you lucky,' she sighs enviously, when her friend is weighed and has lost another two pounds.

'Nothing to do with luck!' I declare. 'She's earned it.'

'Lynn's lucky that she's lost any weight this week, you should just hear about what she ate at McDonalds!' complained Helena.

'Whatever she ate at McDonalds,' I explained, 'she has not eaten to excess over the full week, taking her exercise into account. The whole week's eating counts, not one isolated splurge.' Weight losses are not caused by luck. All weight losses are earned.

I used to envy those folk whose houses were resplendent with luxuriant house plants, lively greenery trailing and sprouting everywhere. My house plants always withered, curled, browned, and died reproachfully.

'Aren't you lucky! Such green fingers!' I used to sigh, enviously. Then I probed the matter further: 'How do you do it?'

'Nothing special,' Mandy replied.

'Well,' disclosed her husband, 'she waters them, she feeds them, she mists those that need misting, she dusts them, she polishes them . . .' Yes. She earns them. No green fingers. She got an instruction book. Read it. Made the effort to carry out the instructions. Succeeded. Just like slimming.

For one of 'my' slimmers it was her second week on the scales, and she had still not lost any weight. Her face showed astonishment.

'Why's this?' I prompted gently. 'You haven't been sticking to your eating guidelines?'

'Well,' she confessed, 'I haven't actually read them yet . . .'

Success: whether it's for beautiful plants or a beautiful-enough body, first read the instructions – all of them! – and make the effort to carry them out.

## COUNTERACT WITH THINK SLIM

- When your thoughts about others' slimming success include the word 'Luck' or 'Lucky', use the Thought-stopping Technique; tell yourself STOP! Check exactly what you are thinking, and think again. It's nothing to do with luck!
- Remind yourself: slimming success is earned.

## YES BUT-ER

She wore a splendid huge hat and an even more huge (but horrendous) navy and white marquee as a guest to the wedding, and when she stood for photos she held her huge white handbag in front of her stomach as if to hide behind it.

'My trouble is that I love my food,' she confided at breakfast the next morning. She wore another marquee, a casual version (if such a thing is possible). I remembered that too-hot, too-fat summer that I wore tents. I had two of them, cool voile with pretty sprigs of Laura Ashley-style flowers. One was lemon; the other pink. I was not cool. I was aware that I looked like a blob of Neapolitan ice cream, and I felt so awkward, hot, tired and old. I was 25.

She had started on the butter on toast whilst she waited for the fry-up.

'Love your food? So do I.' I nodded agreement, drinking my coffee, waiting for my toast.

'Yes, but I *really* love it!' she protested, playing the 'It's Worse for Me than You' game.

'So do I!' I parried, with feeling.

'Yes, but,' she began again, 'you go to work so it's easy for you to avoid the kitchen!'

'Some people's desk drawers are stuffed like a kitchen, with biscuits and crisps,' I started to respond.

'Yes, but it's boring at home!' she complained, carrying on the 'It's Worse for Me than You' theme.

I hadn't learned. I tried again. 'You could get a job.'

'Yes, but I do work part time,' she admitted. 'So I get the worst of both worlds.'

She prattled on, parrying all of my positive suggestions with 'Yes, but . . .' and a thousand and one excuses why no slimming strategy could work for her. She wanted to stay fat and have justification for it. She refused to make the efforts it needs to slim; she was stuck in her fat world and she wanted sympathy, not assistance. She was a 'Yes But-er'.

Yes But-ers have a choice; they can stay overweight and dissatisfied, justifying themselves with their 'Yes, but' game, or they can recognise what they are doing and finally make a choice: to decide to stay fat and accept responsibility for that, and stop plaguing the rest of us; or to stop playing the 'Yes, but' game, accept advice and support, and make the effort it takes to slim.

There is, unfortunately, something of the 'Yes, but' in all of us. We need to notice our 'Yes, buts', smile ruefully at our negative side, and stop the thoughts and sentences that begin with 'Yes but . . .'. Replace them with 'Yes, why not? I'll have a go!'

## COUNTERACT WITH THINK SLIM

- Listen for words and thoughts that begin 'Yes, but' both in others and in yourself. Listening to others helps you to become efficient at picking up the attitude (and you'll be surprised how often it occurs in all sorts of situations).
- Replace, for yourself, 'Yes, but' with 'Yes, Why not? I'll have a go!'

## *THE WISHER*

Willa and her neighbour Dido moved into a new housing estate at about the same time. The builders had left them with uncultivated chaos as gardens, as builders often do. Down the road, some people had moved in twelve months ago, and their garden was resplendent with summer flowers, framed with smooth green grass and dressed with attractive young trees and bushes.

'Ooh, I wish my garden looked like that!' sighed Willa, enviously.

'So do I,' agreed Dido fervently.

Twelve more months went by, and Willa and Dido saw little of each other, as they were both very busy. Soon it was summertime again; and Willa popped round the estate to see Dido. Dido's garden was a picture! Willa was amazed, and envious. Her garden was still a weed-infested, clay-rutted catastrophe.

'Ooh, I wish my garden looked like that!' breathed Willa, jealously.

What was the difference between Willa and Dido? Willa was a Wisher, wishing that her garden would grow, preferably by magic. She would love a nice garden, but she doesn't get round to doing anything to make it happen. Dido was a Do-er. Her wishes became reality because she did something about them.

Slimmers can be Wishers, sighing enviously: 'I wish I was slim . . . I wish I looked like her . . .' but never becoming do-ers. Wishes and dreams are fine; for, in the words of the old song, 'if you don't have a dream, how are you going to have a dream come true?' But wishes are not enough. Plans, plus action, make wishes into reality.

Successful Slimmers *Make* it Happen.

Disastrous Dieters *Let* It Happen.

The only difference between successful slimmers and failures is that the successful ones are do-ers as well as wishers: they plan, act, Think Slim, and persevere.

## COUNTERACT WITH THINK SLIM

- Whenever you see a slim woman that you admire, think: 'I can be like that if I make the effort.'
- Make a Think Slim card(s) with the slogan:

> Successful Slimmers Make It Happen!
> I Can Make It Happen!

## POOR ME!

'I feel so deprived when I'm slimming,' Sally sighed. 'Everyone else in the house is eating everything they want and I can't!'

Deprived. Yes, as slimmers, we are depriving ourselves, but only of some food, for the purpose of getting something else that we want. The Americans call it 'Give Up to Get!' It's a good phrase, for it reminds us that we have chosen to give up one thing, to get something else that we value more.

Opposite to me at a formal dinner sat a woman, piling roast potatoes on to her dish, then over her double chin and into her eager mouth. She wore a blouse billowing over her voluminous Indian-style skirt (which I knew would have an elasticated waist).

'I can't do with all that dieting,' she began, uninvited, to me. That much was obvious from the huge bulk that couldn't be hidden by the tent-like clothes. 'I don't believe in depriving myself of anything!' she declared, decisively.

'Except all the pleasures of being slim,' I reminded her quietly.

She made no answer, but then her mouth was very busy. Busier than her brain, for she had not thought it through.

Consider: who is the more deprived, the slimmer, giving up only some of the foods she loves, but gaining a slim and fit body and all the pleasures that go with it; or, the glutton, over-indulging in every food and drink she/he fancies, but never enjoying the pleasures of living a slim life? I am not suggesting you give up all your favourite foods on a diet. I am teaching you to indulge in your favourite foods, in moderation, within your slimming strategy.

Notice the other words Sally used: 'eating everything they want and *I can't . . .*' Sally's mistaken. She can, if she chooses to. If she chooses to eat everything she wants, she will pay a penalty – she will be overweight. But no one (certainly not me) is telling Sally that she 'can't'. Sally can choose. It's her choice: Everything and be fat. Or, moderation and be slim.

'It's made it so much easier since you said I could have anything I want!' Sally told me, the following week. 'I watch them having chips and I think, well I can have them too, if I want. But I'd rather be slim!'

## COUNTERACT WITH THINK SLIM
- If you are tempted into feeling 'deprived' because you are slimming, use the Thought-stopping Technique. Tell yourself STOP!, and re-think the issue through. Who is more deprived, the slimmer giving up some foods to get what she/he wants (Slim-fitness) or the fattie, eating it all and having it all – all the disadvantages of being overweight and none of the pleasures of a slim-fit lifestyle?
- Think Slim: I'm not deprived. I'm doing what I want to get what I want.
- If anyone asks you: 'can't you have this?'
  Reply: 'I can have what I want, but I've decided not to have it. I'd rather be slim, thank you.'

## THE CINDERS SYNDROME
Cinderella was always my favourite fairy story when I was a child. So romantic: a fairy godmother, all that magic, a beautiful ball gown, a handsome prince – almost lost, except for the glass slipper, and then Living Happily Ever After.

Such are the scripts that are fed into our young heads, lurking there for years to insidiously spoil our slimming years later, when we are grown up (and out). For many slimmers are Cinderellas, waiting for some fairy godmother to come along with magic spells and perform a miracle and transform them from a chubby Cinders to a slim princess. We think we've spotted the fairy godmother in the form of an advertisement: 'send your money for a miracle fat-buster; no dieting, no effort, no exercise.' No chance!

Do you, when you see one of those ads, rush for your cheque book, or maybe think, like Georgia, 'I don't really believe it, but it's tempting, isn't it?' If so, you are still running the Cinderella script in your brain, and you need to switch the off button.

Or maybe you are still playing the Cinders script in your life generally? You'd like a different job, but you'll wait and see if anything turns up. You'd like a boy/girl friend, and it would be nice if one came along. You're tired of how your partner treats you, but you'll hope she/he changes. You'd like to leave your spouse, but you'll see what happens. You'd like some more money, so you'll hope for a rise. You wish your teenage children were more considerate, but that's how they are.

This may sound tough, and it is: but the nearest thing you will get to a fairy godmother is me and this book. Then it is only you who can make it happen. If, like Cinderella, the most active thing you get round to doing about improving your figure and your life is hoping for magic, you will be disappointed.

## COUNTERACT WITH THINK SLIM

- If your slimming is delayed by your pointless search for magic, refuse to delay your slim life any longer. Think Slim: There is *no* magic to get me slim. Only I can make it happen.
- If the Cinders syndrome is the story of the whole of your life, you need to take action to learn to be less passive.

Assertiveness is the quality that will help you; being assertive is about being more confident, knowing what you want, clearly stating your case, and taking action to improve your lot in life rather than waiting for something or someone to rescue you. Assertiveness is an attitude you can acquire and a skill that you can learn to put into practice. (Re-read the earlier pages about assertiveness: 26–30.)

A good first step to take action is to stop and think what you would like to change about your life. Answer these questions both in your thoughts and on paper, considering these areas of your life: work, close relationship, partner, family, social life, hobbies:

1 What am I doing now that I enjoy and still want to do in the future?
2 What am I doing now that I want to do *more* of in the future?
3 What am I doing now that I would like to *stop* doing?
4 What would I like to do instead?
  What would it take to organise it?
  What shall I do next? Short term? Long term?
  When shall I start to do it? (Set dates.)

## NOT ENOUGH TIME
'I've not enough time . . .!'
Actually, we all have exactly the same amount of time. We have 24

hours every 24 hours. We have all the time in the world! That might sound a flippant comment, but it isn't. It's a profound truth that, once accepted, can transform your life. It did mine. For time can be your servant or your master. I read about managing time better, and it isn't only business people who need to learn how to manage their time. It's a skill for everyone who wants to be self-empowered, whether a mum at home with baby, a working man or woman who has to juggle home and work, and for retired people who have extra leisure time to get the most from.

Become a Time Lord. Ask yourself, what exactly is it that you have not enough time for? Often it's the things we are not very keen to do. We always have time to eat our favourite foods. If Richard Gere (or your favourite heart-throb) arrived on your doorstep with an invitation to go to the Caribbean with him/her, on condition you could be changed, washed and packed within one hour, would you have time to get ready? Of course you would!

'Not enough time to get proper meals!' moans Lesley. What she often grabs instead is a succession of chocolate snacks, chips or other fatty take-away fast food. Such snatch and grab habits will soon snatch away your slimming progress, yet all this problem needs is some Think Slim in advance.

The fastest food you can grab for snacks (or for lunch) is fresh fruit.

'But they don't sell it at the petrol station,' grumbles Gill. Does this sound like a 'Yes, but' game coming on? We can't expect life to fall in our laps at the petrol station, or anywhere else. It can become an easy and useful habit to grab a piece of fresh fruit on your way out of the door to be kept in your car in case chaos cancels your planned eating schedule for the day.

Some take-away fast food is amenable to slimming. McDonalds publish a calorie count, and their hamburger is only 252 calories. However, their Big Mac is likely to make a big girl or man of you, with its 552 calories; so will a chocolate milkshake at 388 and large French fries at 385. Yet half a portion of those French fries at 190 calories could be accommodated occasionally – share with a friend. It's simply a matter of choosing wisely.

To James, a proper meal is a hot meal. To all the Jameses out there who think that hot means proper, please think again. Nutritionists tell us that nutrients exist in cold food. In fact, often there is less goodness in hot food, as some of the vitamins and minerals are destroyed by cooking, and/or thrown down the sink with the cooking water. 'Proper' meals, including low-calorie recipes, can be bought in boxes from many good supermarkets; first, check the calories and don't Think Guilt when you open a box or packet. Think Slim: a few minutes with a microwave can save a slimmer's sanity and his/her waistline.

Follow the Earl of Sandwich: a sandwich is a good square meal, if it has no high-fat spread on it. You can buy calorie-laden disasters, but ask in shops that yours be made with no butter or mayonnaise, or buy 'healthy eating' versions from supermarkets. Nutritious and delicious.

Keep a supply of bought sandwiches in the freezer (check their ingredients for freezing suitability) so you have some at the ready. Or, make a stock of your own sandwiches when you have some time (at the weekend?), pack them up in suitable sized pairs and pop them into the freezer.

Your sandwiches will fill and nourish you particularly well if they are accompanied by a pot of my coleslaw recipe (see pages 187–8).

'Not enough time to make up your coleslaw,' Claire objected. Coleslaw is not as interesting as heart-throbs with irresistible invitations, or favourite television programmes, of course. So I got out the ingredients, a sharp knife and a stop-watch, and began to demonstrate how quickly coleslaw can be made.

'Chop it into small chunks, not tiny slivers,' I suggested, 'partly to save time but also to give you more to chew.'

A bowlful was ready in less than three minutes. No time?

'No time to do tummy-crunch exercises!' complained Kelly. No time? You can do three sets of 10, 30 in all, in less than two minutes (see pages 223–4). No time? Or no inclination? Be honest.

My favourite funny-man, Jasper Carrott, made me think again about how I use my time.

He pointed out something like this. If you are 30 years old and live to the proverbial three score years and ten, you have 40 years of living remaining. If you sleep for eight hours each night you will spend 13½ years of the time you have left, asleep; about two years will be spent washing yourself, and three months will disappear while you are using the lavatory! Continue the tale in your own head: there is less time left than you may have assumed – less time, that is, for the pleasurable living that you want to do.

So it's even more important that we check how we are using our time and whether we can use it better. It's terribly true that if you don't use it, you'll lose it.

In 1981, I used to rise, reluctantly and tiredly, after nine and a half hours' sleep, at 8.10 am, and be rushing out of the house just twenty minutes later, at 8.30 – harassed, half asleep, hair awry, always something forgotten. (Nine and a half hours' sleep, in Jasper-speak, is over 15 years of life to a 40 year old.)

'I need my sleep,' I used to declare. 'I'm just not a morning person. I'm one of those people who needs plenty of sleep.' I was wrong.

I changed because I decided that life might be less rushed and more civilised if I dragged myself out of bed, earlier, at 7.45; also I decided to buy an exercise bike. To 'get on me bike' needed more time.

Surprise, surprise, I didn't suffer from exhaustion due to lack of sleep. I exercised, and actually felt almost human by 8.30. Then I tried alarming myself for 7.30; then 7.15 (and wasn't that a struggle at first!) and so could include 20 minutes on the bike.

Then Dixie the Dog came into my life; bred to win show prizes, she was rejected by her first owners because she wasn't perfect enough. She fits me – and my un-perfect philosophy of life – fine. But Dixie's bounding body needed to be walked. Now, I had always thought of 6.45 am as the middle of the night, but I have learned that it's not too difficult to change my thoughts. So I decided to get up at 6.45 am so I could perform the dog-walk chore.

The great news is that it's not a chore. Dixie and I make our harmonious, unperfect way round the woods, and I've found beauty and peace and time to put my all-important thoughts in order for the day. It took even more change in my thinking to accept a 6.30 reveille, but I thought to myself that there's no use wasting my life asleep. 'Practising for dead' is what I call it now.

Then, I changed my job; an earlier start and a longer journey demanded an earlier routine, so now, I'm awakened at 5.45. To me, the amazing and wonderful thing about it is that I am no more tired than I was, years younger, awaking at 8.10. I have just under seven hours' sleep a night nowadays.

I have discovered for myself what the sleep experts tell us, that our 'sleep needs' are largely a matter of habit. Maybe there is a necessary minimum, and that most of us need seven to eight hours' sleep – or maybe we don't.

I'm delighted to tell you and Jasper Carrott that I've knocked off two hours a night sleep, and gained almost an extra day each week to spend living!

## COUNTERACT WITH THINK SLIM
- We limit ourselves by what we think; probably all you need is a change of your thoughts; Think Slim: 'I've got 24 hours every 24 hours. I can decide what to do with them.'
- Review, honestly, how you spend your time. (Don't be tempted into defending yourself with how marvellously busy you are already – everyone can improve their use of time.) Start by analysing your habits, and use the following tips:

  1 Analysis. Ask yourself:

  How much time do I waste? With what? Or with whom?

  How much time is spent on unnecessary household chores? (such as ironing underwear, socks, towels, sheets: making cupboard-contents look like rows of soldiers).

  How much time is wasted clearing up after others who are perfectly capable of clearing up their own muddle? When are you going to insist that they do it (or find their belongings in a pile outside the house)?

  2 Time Saving Tips:

  Live by lists. Make lists so that things are not forgotten, are done in the quickest order, and no extra journeys are incurred.

Prioritise your jobs so that you do not hassle yourself with overrun deadlines.

Do two things at once. Have some easy job on hand while you watch television, or tackle telephone calls (they inevitably involve waiting time; buy a hands-free phone if you can afford to change).

Have little spare jobs, or lists to write, or papers/books to read if you have any 'Waiting Time' imposed on you (at bus stops, train stations, when travelling by bus, train, as a car passenger, or by aeroplane).

Read a book about time management. (Resist making jokes about how you've no time to read it!) Read it whilst pedalling on your exercise bike – saves time!

## THE URGE

'I was fine all week and then last night, I got home after my badminton game and I had this terrible urge to eat!' moaned Carolyn, exasperated with herself. 'Then I started and I ate a whole malt loaf! And now I've not lost any weight!'

'The Urge' is familiar to many slimmers. It has two main causes.

### 1  TOO LITTLE FOOD DURING THE DAY

All day you have starved your body, yet made demands on it for the energy to go to work, rush to the shops, walk the dog, romp with the baby, do the housework. You are feeling virtuous and clever and very in control – and that's all because you are still trapped by diet-think. Diet-think that preaches (wrongly) that denying yourself food all day is being 'good', and the less eaten the 'better' you have been.

'I can go all day hardly eating anything. Then, wham, I get this dreadful urge and in no time I've eaten cakesful of calories!'

Is it any wonder that you get this dreadful urge? Your body is demanding, very loudly and rightly, that you stop this cruel starvation and give it the food it needs. Why should we be so cruel to ourselves? Would you treat your dog like that?

Ivana Trump is reputed to have said that when she is hungry she feels powerful. How sad that she needs to go hungry to feel powerful. I should like Ivana, and all slimmers, to feel powerful (self-empowered and secure) all of the time without any need to starve themselves. Some experts also believe that anorexics are looking for and need a feeling of power (that they otherwise lack in their lives), when they are controlling their intake of food and their body weight.

Our bodies are part of ourselves, not a thing apart to be starved and battered by neglect and deliberate torture. Re-think your attitude to your body. It is an intrinsic part of you and, let's face it, a pretty remarkable creation. Be kind to both your body and yourself – every human being deserves that.

## COUNTERACT WITH THINK SLIM

- Remember that your body is part of yourself, and deserves your consideration.
- Think 'Kind' to yourself and to your body.
- We all need to feel self-empowered, and there are many ideas in this book to help you achieve that in more helpful ways than starving yourself. (See Step One, page 17.)
- Recognise that your body is like a car that needs fuel – good, sensible food – to start and to work.
- Give your body regular 'fuel' by spacing your meals regularly.
- Nourish your body by the sorts of food that you choose. (Step Six, page 167, explains how.)
- Take a one-a-day vitamin and mineral tablet, because those on less than 3000 calories of varied food per day are unlikely to take in all the vitamins and minerals they need.

## 2 'THE URGE' AND OUR EMOTIONS

The second main cause of 'the Urge' is that we have an emotional hole to fill, which we are not aware of, and so we re-route this, subconsciously, into an urge to eat. This appears to be a reaction found in women more than men.

'How were you feeling at the time you got The Urge?' I asked Carolyn.

'I don't know,' she replied.

'Try to think,' I encouraged her.

She pondered, but did not know.

Unfortunately, we often 'don't know' how we are feeling. This is true of both men and women, although there are differences in their upbringings that result in different approaches to feelings.

Women, generally, are brought up to express caring feelings; caring for others, that is, before or instead of themselves. For women it is acceptable also to express tears and sorrow, worry and anxiety (again, especially about other people); and depression is commonly expressed by females. What women are taught to suppress is anger, particularly in respect of how they themselves are being treated. It is OK to get angry about starving orphans abroad, but to feel and show anger about your own situation in life, about the man or family who take you for granted is not so acceptable. We learn this lesson very young, with the result that we block off the feelings so efficiently that we do not know how we feel. All we know is that we want to eat.

Samantha told how, one Sunday morning, she was cleaning upstairs after breakfast, and was feeling fine. Coming downstairs she suddenly felt 'The Urge'.

'I could just murder a piece of toast,' she thought. 'I must have a piece of toast!'

Fortunately, she was learning to Think Slim.

'Why?' she thought. 'Why have I got that sudden urge?'

She didn't know. But she stood still and thought: 'Trace it back. I was

OK cleaning upstairs. Then what happened? Oh, yes, the phone rang. My husband called up to tell me his parents would be over to see us later. That's it! That's what has bothered me. I said, OK. But it isn't OK. They are often calling on us without earlier notice and we are so busy because we both go to work. I realised that I felt angry and resentful, that I should have to go and smile and be pleasant and I'd be fuming inside. That's why I got The Urge for toast.'

When she recognised her feelings, The Urge disappeared. The anger didn't, but now at least she knew what was wrong, and she and her husband could probably gently explain to the parents that they loved to have them visit, but needed to know in advance.

Sometimes we may know that we are feeling angry, but still get The Urge. Diane explained: 'that awful woman at the committee meeting! I was so cross with her, and didn't like to say anything. I came home and ate and ate . . .!'

Diane needs to be more assertive with awful women at committee meetings. Or, if the committee meeting is always a hassle, perhaps she should consider resigning. Who needs such hassle? This is Not A Dress Rehearsal. Diane could do other things.

Eating is no helpful antidote to anger. I know it works, for a few seconds. But it makes us fat. We need other, more useful ways of dealing with our feelings. If we are angry our body is aroused and we need to dissipate that energy. Activity can help. Walk fast, dig the garden, pound a pillow, cycle, dance around. Then relax.

The Urge may not be due to anger-feelings. It may be caused by a desire for comfort. Somehow, you know you can depend on chocolate, while you're not sure of your spouse or your best friend.

'My washing machine broke down, and there was water all over the floor . . .' and I ate two pieces of sponge cake!' explained Jay.

She may have done better to use the sponge cake to soak up some of the water!

'I'd had a bad day, having to be nice to unreasonable customers,' was Alison's reason for comforting herself with a few chocolate biscuits.

'Well, I deserve this' is the downfall thought of many a slimmer, as emotional eating – for comfort or reward – adds excess calories and excess pounds to the day.

'I've had problems,' began Sian, waving her hand expressively round her bulging body, 'and it shows.'

Her problems were with the man in her life. Sian thinks that he'll change for the better, that if only she does this, or that, he'll reform. He drinks too much but promises to give up, and she thinks, 'maybe this time'. She thinks it must be awful to be alone, so she accepts the unacceptable from him, and eats, and gets fatter. Her thoughts are not rational. It does not have to be awful to be alone. (I lived as a single parent for six years. I thought it peaceful.) It will only be awful if you insist on thinking it awful. You cannot change the behaviour of the man in your life unless he sees the need for it and is willing.

If you are willing to play the doormat, there will be people prepared to walk over you. Respect yourself; refuse to accept the unacceptable. If the man in your life doesn't treat you how you want to be treated, tell him so, tell him what you want, and be prepared to leave if he refuses. This is not a Dress Rehearsal.

Do not suffer in silent comfort-eating. For, it is not possible to eat yourself happy. You can only eat yourself fat. Yes, for a few moments, you can feel comforted by food, but food, like drugs, has unwanted side-effects – it makes you fat. It's a sad fact of life that we cannot have the food without having its side-effects. So, we have to choose.

There are other ways of getting comfort. Favourite comforting music. Favourite, perfumed, bath foam works for me. Or, if you want attention from another person – *go and ask for it*. Unashamedly, ask.

'You can't ask . . .!' people often say, incredulously. Why not? It's healthier than eating. (Some people do more than eat: some women turn to tranquillisers, men turn to violence.)

'I want a cuddle,' I say to my husband. Say what *you* want.

Men, too.

'I don't show my feelings, me,' he declared, speaking the macho script that he has been taught all his life, 'except anger, of course.'

Of course. Boys will be boys and boys are allowed to be angry. Anger is real-men emotion.

Men need to rid themselves of this cultural conditioning that burdens them with aggressive tendencies and a stiff upper lip. Men, too, need to get in touch with the whole range of their feelings, and recognise when they need comfort.

Men, generally, don't so much comfort-eat as comfort-drink. Off down to the local to drown the sorrows they can't speak, but alcohol is calorie-loaded (about 100 calories for half a pint/300 ml of beer) so this choice of tranquilliser is very fattening.

Men, too, could ask for the comfort they need, talk over their worries about money, work, sex or whatever, with their partner or a friend. Or even with a professional counsellor. John Cleese, the humorist, took professional psychotherapy and has since written it into a book and radio series. It might even enhance your business, as it did his.

## COUNTERACT WITH THINK SLIM
- Think: It is OK to have feelings and to pay attention to them.
- If you get The Urge and don't know why, trace back your feelings and the events of the day so far.
  Ask: When did I start to feel The Urge?
      What was I thinking about?
      What had happened?
      Was I all right earlier?
Keep going back until you trace what triggered The Urge. Something did. As you do this more often, it becomes easier to find the trigger,

and you can then plan how to avoid it, or deal with it better in the future.

- Think Slim: Food can't solve problems. Only I can do that. More food simply means more fat.

## NOT FAIR

'It's Not Fair! My husband can eat everything in sight yet he's really skinny and never puts on a pound!' Diana moans.

'And that woman in Personnel – she's the same!' joins in Shirley.

Everyone knows someone who can eat all they want and still stay slim. And we all hate them. Me, too. It certainly is not fair. But, then, life isn't fair. Did anyone ever promise you that it would be? I'm afraid not.

We can do nothing about those extra-fortunate people who can eat to their mind's content; if you can't bear to be with them, don't be friends with them, and don't choose to marry them! It cannot help us to stamp our feet and sulk and console ourselves with another cream cake, just because it is not fair.

We could usefully be guided by the prayer of Alcoholics Anonymous: 'change what can be changed, and have the grace to accept that which cannot be changed'. You can cultivate such grace by repeating in your thoughts that: 'OK I accept that life is never going to be fair.'

After all, maybe it also isn't fair that we were born in countries where food is so plentiful that we can over-eat so easily, while much of the world is starving. So, maybe we are the lucky ones.

### COUNTERACT WITH THINK SLIM

- Think: 'OK, it isn't fair. *Life* isn't fair. I accept it.'
- Stop yourself being a Moan-A-Lot; Count your blessings – it's we who are the lucky ones.

## THE DEMON IMPS

There are two 'Demon Imps' which often invade our thoughts and sabotage our slimming. The Demons are IMPatience and IMPulse.

### THE DEMON IMP – IMPATIENCE

By when do we want to be slim? Tomorrow morning – at the latest! The Demon Imp whispers in our mind and demands impossibly quick results. So we often fall for the lure of the 'quick fix' diet: the banana and milk diet, the Very Low Calorie Diets, the 'Lose seven pounds in seven days' (3 kilos) regimes; we lose weight (probably still not quickly enough to satisfy our Demon Imp), but promptly put it back on again.

'Only two pounds lost,' screeches Mae in disappointment, at the scales. It's an excellent weight loss (about 1 kilo), but the Demon Imp in ourselves is dissatisfied.

'All that effort for only two pounds,' complains Dinah's Demon. Then she feels demoralised; maybe a donut or three will comfort her.

'If I haven't lost weight this week, I'm giving up!' threatens Lisa. There's the Demon again, too impatient to accept our body's own rhythm, as it adjusts to our slimming. Sometimes there is a 'plateau' when our efforts are the same as before but the weight loss doesn't happen. Sometimes that plateau must be endured, and we must silence our own Demon Imp.

Research indicates that in Britain, about 50 per cent of people who start slimming have given up within a month, victims of their own Demon Impatience. Such impatience is encouraged by our culture's emphasis on 'Instantism'. Not so long ago, there was an advertising campaign by a world-wide company of slimming groups which lured with a 'Quick-start' Programme. To re-read 'Instantism' in Negative Wizards and our culture see page 57.

## COUNTERACT WITH THINK SLIM

- Think of *realistic* targets of weight loss, to average no more than between one or two pounds (half to one kilo) per week. (See Step 3: Target Yourself, page 127.)
- If ever you find yourself beset by thoughts from your Demon Impatience, use the Thought-stopping Technique: tell yourself 'Stop This!' and replace it with 'I'm doing fine. I'm on the right track.'
- If you lose half a pound/quarter of a kilo of weight in one week, you could do as Julia does – announce to yourself '8 oz lost'/'250 grammes lost' instead; she thinks it sounds a better result and she feels more encouraged by it.
- Think forward and set a (*realistic*) long-term target as well as short ones. This reminds you that you are starting a long-term project, not a quick-fix.
- Notice cultural advertisements which encourage impatience in slimming ('Lose 7 lb in 7 Days' etc) and scoff at them.
- Remind yourself that weight lost quickly is often weight regained quickly; slower loss gives your body time to re-adjust and gives you time to learn a different, permanent style of slim-living.

## THE DEMON IMP – IMPULSE

Rational thinking – and slimming – can go out of the window when the Demon Impulse intrudes on our lives. The Demon Impulse whispers its seductive thoughts, and, too often, we succumb to its tempting words. Impulse can spoil slimming in three different situations:

1 **Eating on impulse.** 'Just one won't hurt.' (But it won't be 'one', will it?)

'I'll take the large economy pack of fun-size choc bars, they'll last longer.' (But one fun-size leads to another, and another . . .)

'I'll have it now and make up for it tomorrow!' (But tomorrow never comes.)

Many a hundred calories are swallowed, on impulse, before we have really considered whether we want to eat. Swallowed, also, almost before it is tasted.

**2 Starting slimming on impulse.** 'Right, that's it!' we declare, one day, when skirt after skirt has been discarded as too tight and we are left with nothing to wear. 'I'm starting to slim, from this very minute!'

Yet, starting to slim, impulsively in this way, is not always a good thing, not without thinking it through and planning. To achieve slimming success, it is necessary to decide realistically what we are aiming for, and just how we shall achieve it. This book guides you through that very process, and helps to ensure that you don't reel from one poor impulse to the next.

**3 Finishing slimming on impulse.** 'Oh, blow it, I've had enough of this slimming business,' we fume impulsively, as we are faced with another frustrating day, only a tiny weight loss on the scales, and cream cakes in the coffee shop. The cream cakes are swallowed, and so is our determination and all hope of becoming slimmer. The cause of our downfall was our habit of thinking impulsively and acting on that impulse.

How to Defeat the Demon? In all of the situations just described, the answer to the threat of the Demon Impulse is to Stop, and Think. Think Slim. Before we act – and eat – we need to Think, rationally and honestly, about what we are about to do, and why.

'Oh,' do I hear you moan, as I've heard other slimmers, 'do we have to do all this thinking?'

Sometimes true answers are ones that we don't want to hear; tough answers. The tough truth is that all this thinking is necessary (and thinking is hard work!). However, we do 'think' daily in other areas of our life; for example when crossing the road. We don't grumpily decide that it's too much effort to think, and walk across without looking. If we did, a big bus or careering car would make mincemeat of us. Similarly, if we don't Think before we eat, the Demon Impulse will surely make fat of us.

## COUNTERACT WITH THINK SLIM
- Think Slim: I Think Before I Eat.
- Think Slim when faced by any item of food: is it worth its calories?
- Make a Think Slim Card:
  Do I really Want it?
  No I don't.
  Shall I eat it?
  No, I won't!
Carry the Think Slim card around with you, or put it in a spot most convenient for reminding you. Or make a few cards, to be kept in

different places. (Impulse is a very persistent saboteur; in a survey of my slimming groups, this Negative Wizard was the most commonly reported one.)

- Make a Food and Drink Diary (there is a sample sheet in the Appendix of this book, see page 263). Write down what you are about to eat, just *before* you eat it (not after). If you change your mind about eating it, simply cross it off. (Your diary is yours and it does not have to be neat.) Check the weight of your portions (guessing means overweight – both the portion and you). Carry the diary around with you everywhere: filling it in *before* you eat ensures that you stop to think, and the Negative Wizard Impulse loses its power.

  Many of my slimmers find that such a Diary is one of their best aids to success. Sara explains: 'It's made me think, and I've weighed my portions, and I've lost 2½ pounds/1 kilo this week for the first time in ages. It's really worth the effort.'

- Take some time to consider what Impulsive mistakes you have made, and how you cope better in the future using Think Slim principles. Write down examples of your Impulsive past mistakes, and ideas for future coping:

**Impulsive Mistakes**          **Think Slim Ideas for Future Coping**

......................................................................................................................

......................................................................................................................

......................................................................................................................

......................................................................................................................

......................................................................................................................

## *BEING MRS GOODWIFE*

Marriage can fatten your figure! Or, rather, playing at being Mrs Goodwife can.

'I wanted to prove what a good wife I was, with lots of good food, a good home, and everything just right!' explains Hannah.

The Food of Love: giving him food is seen as giving him love. Knee high, women are taught that 'the way to a man's heart is through his stomach'. But by 'good food' Hannah, like others, means high-calorie cakes, pies, puds and desserts. Women's magazines are full of calorific recipes which she is not-so-subtly pressured to produce for him and the family. But it is no way to be a good wife, providing him with a heart attack on a plate, making him overweight, pushing up his blood pressure, and caking up his arteries with cholesterol. (Unless, of course, your aim is to become a merry, slim widow.) If you want to give love, give love. Don't wrap it up in calories.

A woman's place is in the danger zone. Being in the kitchen, cooking and experimenting, can be a new and extra food-temptation for a young wife whose (overweight) mum used to be the one to do that.

When cooking, food 'tasting' can become a habit – a lifelong, fattening habit. Jeanne had been making gravy successfully for the 25 years she had been married, but she still always tasted it (liberally), kidding herself that she needed to check that it's just right. Jeanne kicked the habit and went on to lose all her 2 stones/13 kilos of excess weight. Him Indoors was delighted and bought her some fuschia French knickers – and he still likes the (untasted) gravy.

Being a good wife who eats with him, in intimate togetherness, just like him, in the same quantities as he does, is another common mistake. I used to do that. But, men's bodies naturally require more food than women's, partly because of the obvious reason that men are usually taller and larger than women, but also because men were given greater muscle mass than women. Muscle burns up more calories than fat (a point in favour of exercising your body into a more muscled version) so men can, generally, eat more than women. This is even more true if he's a rugby-playing six-footer, and she's a five-foot-nothing non-sportswoman whose idea of exercise is wrestling to unwrap a packet of biscuits.

Now, I accept there's no equality on the dinner plates. I started to use a smaller plate for me, to console myself and make my portion look bigger. Today, I'm more realistic and accepting: same size plate, less food, slim me.

The pressures of getting everything 'just right', even when you have a job and/or a young child to care for, is liable to turn many a wife's fancy to foodie comforts.

It is not possible to Do-It-All. Nor should we attempt to try. Ideal homes should stay where they belong, on magazine pages, not in our minds to try to achieve. 'Everything OK' is plenty good enough, with both you and he taking equal responsibility for keeping it that way. He won't? What you mean is, that *you allow him not to*.

Perhaps you like him dependent on you – it makes you feel safe, believing that he won't leave you. Doing-It-All to feel safe is not worth it. For you can never be that safe, and you simply have to live with the fear. Besides, if you're so shattered from Doing-It-All, slumping around, overweight and irritable, he might well start straying towards slim and sociable women.

You swear it, he won't help? You've tried everything, including leaving this page open for him to read? Then, write to me for the name of a good divorce lawyer. There are millions of other men out there, and it's better to check out their attitudes before you say anything like 'I do'.

## COUNTERACT WITH THINK SLIM
- Think Slim: There is no need to 'play Mrs Goodwife'.

If I want to give love, I'll give love not food.

There is no need to Do-It-All.

There is no need for everything to be just right – everything OK is plenty good enough.

- Housework: do as little as possible in the shortest possible time, and make sure others in the household do their share. (You could read Shirley Conran's book *Down With Superwoman* for tips, including how to get the others to do their share.)

## THE SECRET EATER

The three of us always ate in the company dining room together. We all ate careful salads. Two of us were slim. She was a size 24 salad-eater. She always protested her innocence. She ate like a bird, just like us, but her metabolic rate must be so pathetic that it caused her to be a size 24 on size 10 eating habits.

She didn't fool me, because I've been a secret eater, wide-eyed with public innocence and private guilt. Then one day, she confided to me that after the dining room salad, she went home and ate again.

Eating in secret is very common. Sal had a dressing gown with big pockets, to hide her chocolate bars. Vi ate her Mars Bars in the bath, so no one could hear the noise of the paper rustling. Jackie often woke during the night, so she sneaked off down to raid the fridge for cheese.

Why do we eat in secret? Often it is because we are stuck in diet-think. We think we are not entitled to any of our favourite high-calorie foods, and we feel guilty about being overweight and about our eating. But we crave our favourites (naturally, being denied them) so off we sneak. Or, we are emotional eaters, hoping that food will heal the hurt, or soothe the anger, or lift the depression. (If this seems to be like you, read the Negative Wizards section on The Urge again, page 80.)

Secret eating is no help. As my husband once said to me: it is just as fattening if you eat it in secret.

So, it adds to your weight, but also does other damage: it prompts guilt, it inveigles you into deceiving others and telling lies, and so it saps your self-respect and your confidence. As your self-respect and confidence plummet, your slimming slips further into failure.

### COUNTERACT WITH THINK SLIM

- Remember: with this slim-fit slimming system, you can include your favourite foods. Eat them (in moderation!) in public, without guilt and with enjoyment. Jenny followed this advice, and her husband remarked: 'I know you're serious about slimming this time. You don't close the door any more when you go into the kitchen!' Jenny's jaunts to the kitchen had always been for secret eating. No more. No more excess 5 stones/32 kilos in weight, either.
- Think Slim: It's Just As Fattening If You Eat it In Secret!' You may fool the public, but you can't fool the scales.

## THAT LI'L BIT

'If I haven't lost weight this week, it must be your scales!' shrieks Lil.

She hasn't lost weight and she can't understand it. Tears of frustration and anger sting at her eyes, and she blinks them back. Lil is absolutely certain that she has stuck to her eating programme. She planned her meals carefully, and nothing extra went on her plate. But let's check out what actually happened, one day in the life of Lil.

Sunday morning: she starts with her breakfast cereal, but she tips it enthusiastically into her bowl. 'Good slimming food, this,' she thinks. 'Everybody knows that.' She thinks there's no need to measure out good slimming food. Her Programme's 1 ounce/28 grammes of cereal falls into her bowl as 3. An extra 200 calories.

Later, she clears away the table. Her tiny terror, three-year-old Benjamin, has, as usual, left the crusts from his very buttery, jammy toast. Absent-mindedly, Lil pops the crusts into her mouth instead of the bin. (Seventy calories.) She thinks that it's a disgrace to waste good food when there are millions starving in the world. Everybody thinks that, don't they?

Elevenses. Not for Lil, of course. Just for Benjamin. A biscuit. (Children have to have biscuits and Good Mothers have to provide them, Lil thinks.) There's a few of those biscuits at the bottom of the tin, broken ones, and no Good Mother can give those to a child, so where do they go? Yes, into Lil. 'That Li'l Bit won't hurt,' she thinks happily. (One hundred calories.)

As any good wife should, she's cooking Sunday Lunch. Proper Sunday Lunch. Roast beef, vegetables, roast potatoes (not that she's having any of those); proper puddings for the family – a choice of Lil's home-made apple pie with cream, or jam sponge with custard (not that she's having any of those). But good wives have to provide proper puddings for the family, thinks Lil.

She tastes the gravy, only because you have to check it's good enough for the family, you understand. A dessertspoon. Another 50 calories. She serves out the roast potatoes; none for her, of course. Some of the bits are stuck at the bottom of the dish, and she digs at them with her spatula, and pops them into her mouth. 'That Li'l Bit won't hurt!' she thinks. But those bits are the most fatty, at least 200 calories lurking in them.

The family eat their proper puddings, but not Lil. She has a low fat yoghurt – oh yes, and a lick of the cream carton and a finger lickin' of the custard jug. 'That Li'l Bit won't . . .' she thinks. Another 75 calories.

It is a lazy Sunday afternoon. Lil is sunbathing while Benjamin runs around. It's too hot for Lil to run around. Benjamin fetches the sweeties his Good Grandmother has bought for him and pushes one politely at Mum. Only a boiled sweet. You really can't refuse a polite little child, can you? And That Li'l Bit . . . Another 50 calories.

Lil hears a bell; it reminds her of the bell that's rung in her slimming group when someone reaches their target of weight loss. 'Bet I'll never be that lucky,' Lil thinks. The bell is from the mobile ice-cream van.

Benjamin wants. Benjamin gets. Lil has to carry back the cornet to the garden, for it's already melting, and she has to give it a saving lick, or two. Thick vanilla ice cream. Another few calories; only 25. That Li'l Bit . . .

Dinner-time is slimming food again for her – salad. As for Benjamin's sandwich crusts, well of course he leaves them and they go the way of all left-overs. Into Lil. Well, it's disrespectful to waste good food and That Li'l Bit . . . Another 60 calories.

Lil's husband Joe suggests they pop to the pub for a quick one; it's such a lovely evening and they can sit outside with Benjamin. 'Mineral water for me,' says Lil, virtuously. Benjamin wants crisps. Benjamin gets. He offers some to mum, who thinks you can't refuse a child; and it is, after all, only a Li'l Bit. Another 30 calories.

Some friends arrive and join them.

'No thank you, no peanuts and only a mineral water,' calls Lil.

He offers peanuts to Lil, as any polite friend would.

'No thanks,' she replies determinedly.

'Oh, go on, Lil. That li'l bit won't hurt,' he encourages.

'Of course it won't,' thinks Lil, and holds out her hand. Peanuts tend to erupt from a packet in a rush, and a peanut or two become nine. $9 \times 5 = 45$. Forty-five calories.

Lil goes to bed that night contentedly. She thinks she has done really well today with her slimming. She followed all her eating guidelines. 'This week,' she thinks, delightedly, 'I shall have lost at least two pounds, maybe even more!'

How many extra calories did Lil have, over and above her day's allowance in her meals? A massive 705. Extra. She thinks that she had 1000 calories today, but in fact she devoured 1705. No wonder Lil hasn't lost weight. If she did this very often, she would put *on* weight – and still be blaming the scales.

## COUNTERACT WITH THINK SLIM
- Make yourself aware of everything that goes into your mouth. Think before you eat a thing.
- Make a Think Slim card: 'Think Before You Eat a Thing.'
- Remember that every calorie counts. Even if you forget it, the scales won't.
- Measure out your portions, especially cereal. There is no such thing as 'slimming food'. All food fattens if you don't work it off. Some food is less fattening than others, but don't fall into the think-trap that some food is 'good slimming food'.
- Avoid the think-trap of 'what about the starving millions?' which leads you to eat the left-overs. It cannot help the starving millions if you eat up left-overs and get fat; they will still be starving. If you care about the starving millions, do something practical about raising money for them. Think Slim, repeatedly: 'It can't help the starving millions if I eat left-overs and get fat.'

- Think whether you are often cooking too much, and if so, cut down.
- Think of a plan for what to do with left-overs. Into the bin; into the birds; into a family pet (but not too much or it will get fat); into the fridge to use later; or into the freezer to use another day. Think it through and decide now.
- As soon as you start to prepare meals, put a bowl of hot sudsy water ready for the bowls to be immersed in immediately, before they are finger-licked.

## FAT HABITS
Habits: 'At first cobwebs . . . at last chains.'

(Old proverb)

You always have a biscuit (or three) with your coffee.

Always have cheese and biscuits just before bed.

Always buy a bar of chocolate with your newspaper, your petrol, your weekly shop.

Always sneak downstairs to raid the fridge if you can't sleep.

Habits increase in strength, the longer we keep them. The good news is that they can be replaced with habits more helpful to our slimming, and these Slim Habits become as strong as our Fat Habits did.

I used to have a bag of chocolate eclair sweets every Saturday morning, bought with my bread. It was a difficult habit for me to break then. Yet, I had since forgotten that I ever had such a habit until recently something jolted my memory about it. My Saturday sweet habit was over ten years ago; nowadays my mind never goes to sweets on a Saturday morning. Sweets on Saturdays is not part of my life anymore, and I'm not more miserable because of it – I am more slim!

'I always nibbled when I was watching television, admitted Sonia. 'Now, for the last three weeks I haven't done it at all and I feel OK about it now.'

Stella always had a goodie bag of crisps and nuts on Friday evenings when she and her husband settled down to watch a video. It's a habit she's now broken and her slimming is benefiting.

Human beings are creatures of habit. Habit can be useful because it makes life easier. If you do something once, it is likely that you will do it again. If you do something 20 times, you'll probably do it 2000 times. However, when the habit is a fattening one, it's another saboteur.

A famous psychologist, Pavlov, experimented with dogs, ringing a bell when he fed them. Naturally, the dogs salivated over the food. Then, after a while, he rang the bell without producing any food, and the dogs still salivated at the sound of the bell. They were associating the bell sound with food, and their bodies reacted as if food was there. In a sense, we are all like Pavlov's dogs; associating certain things with food, and craving the food we associate. So that cup of coffee brings on the association of biscuit; the night-time awakening associates with the food in the fridge; and so on.

We need to break those associations. At first it may be difficult, and saying no to yourself may not stop the craving. If the craving is there, do something else to occupy your mind, for it is really impossible to think of two things at once. If you give in to the craving occasionally, it's a good idea to tell yourself: 'OK, I'll have this but I will wait five minutes before I eat it.' Then wait, do something else, even if it's only to go and wash your hands. This puts you in control, making your own decision, and you are not the totally helpless victim of your craving.

When I had chocolate cravings at work at lunch-time, I used to promise myself 'I won't have it now but I can have it tomorrow'. Mostly, by tomorrow, the craving had disappeared and I could do without it.

Persevere in getting rid of your fat habits. If you lapse, try again.

## COUNTERACT WITH THINK SLIM
- Think about the fattening habits that you need to change. Write them down and set about changing them, one at a time. (Don't tackle them all at once if there is a long list.)
- It is better to replace a habit with something else to do, if possible.
- If you lapse into your old habit, don't assume you've failed and give up; be patient with yourself. If you've had a habit for a long time, it may take a time to break. Just start again, determined to break the habit.

## THE NEGA-THINKER
'It's so miserable, slimming!' sighs Nega-thinker.

'I can't be bothered with checking the calories!' she grumbles.

'It's such a drag having to weigh food portions!' she moans.

'It takes so long to slim . . .'

'All this thinking about everything is such a bore . . .'

Nega-thinker accentuates the negative. She makes herself – and everyone around her – more negative, more miserable, and more likely to fail at slimming.

I used to be a Nega-thinker, wallowing in my moans and 'Can't-bee's'. My inspiration was a woman called Pam I became friends with, who amazed me with her cheerful 'no problem' response to all the world.

'Could you two manage . . . ?' Before I could scoff in my cynical way, 'You must be joking!', she'd answered for us: 'Yeah, fine. No problem.' What was even more amazing was that we always did manage it, no problem. Believing it was the essential step to completing it.

Being friends with Positive Pam changed me, as I, too, began to respond like her. It will work for you, too. The Positive Attitude makes successful action. If you decide you will *do* something, then you can decide *how*. *How* is about planning.

Catch your nega-thoughts. What are you thinking that's negative? I checked on myself and found that I used to think, repeatedly: 'Oh, I can't be bothered,' and whatever it was would not be done. Even small things, like taking a garment upstairs, or filing away a letter; jotting down a date. Can't be bothered to weigh the portion; can't be bothered to make up some coleslaw.

The 'can't be bothered' habit leads to chaos and slimming failure. It saps your self-confidence as chaos piles up around you, as does the fat. You feel even less effective, and even more 'can't be bothered'.

You can change this successfully by monitoring your thoughts. For example, whenever I caught myself thinking 'I can't be bothered' I replaced it with 'yes, I can – I'll do it now!' This has made a tremendous difference to my life, and it can to yours. You will be more successful at your slimming and also with your life generally. Things get done; things happen. Successful slimmers make it happen; disastrous dieters let it happen.

### COUNTERACT WITH THINK SLIM
- Accentuate the positive, never the negative: 'I'm solving my weight problem. OK, it's taking some time, but I'm solving it!'
- Refuse to join in a Nega-thinker game with other slimmers.
- Monitor your own thinking to find out what nega-thoughts are sabotaging you. Think of a positive alternative to always replace the negative one. All your responses become a habit, so, habitually change moans of 'It can't be done' to 'OK, I'll do it'.
- Cultivate the Pollyanna attitude – optimistic and cheerful.
- 'No Problem' is useful Think Slim. (You could print it on your T-shirt as well as in your thoughts and on your lips.)

## NOT AT MY AGE!

'Perhaps I'm too old to bother,' whispered Annie tentatively, the first time she arrived at my slimming group.

'Of course you're not,' I smiled encouragingly, 'you're *never* too old to bother. "Bothering" is what makes life worth living.'

Annie, sixty-something, went on to lose over 2 stones/13 kilos in weight.

The famous forty-something actor, Jack Nicholson, is reported as saying: 'At my age you can't expect to see your toes.' Whether or not Tom, Jack or Harriet can see those toes is not a function of age, but it may well be a matter of expectations. If we 'expect' not to see our toes simply because we are older, we won't bother to slim and to exercise; our expectations will come true because we make no efforts.

A reader recently wrote to a slimming magazine, lamenting that it never shows successful 'Before and After' stories of older women, of similar age to herself. The editor, quite rightly, pointed out that many such stories did appear regularly. I knew that was true, for I read and save such stories.

Why hadn't this older reader noticed them? Psychology studies indicate that human beings have an unfortunate tendency to notice evidence that supports the ideas they already have, and to ignore evidence to the contrary. This 'selective' way of viewing the world makes our life easier and us more comfortable, as we are not shaken out of our cherished beliefs. But it leaves us stuck in a prejudiced thought-rut and in old habits, too. Sometimes, such thoughts and habits keep us fat.

That older, overweight reader had her fat and had her excuse too, while enjoying her over-eating and not bothering to exercise. She, maybe subconsciously, didn't want to see older people successfully slimming (or she would lose her comfortable excuse), so she didn't notice them. We can choose what to focus on. I focus on good role models of older people, so I don't worry about getting older.

I collect pictures and stories of older people who inspire me; one of my favourites is of keep-fitter Margaret Morris, working out in Regent's Park, wearing a bikini, at 75 years of age. Another is of a 91-years-young ex-Tiller Girl dancer showing her still-high kick. 'Stars' such as Tina Turner, Joan Collins and Raquel Welch demonstrate the possibilities. Mary Wesley's novels were first published when she was 70; Hannah Hauxwell (at 65) writes her stories of her Yorkshire country life into the British best-sellers; George Burns, the American comedian, still wisecracks his way through his nineties; Norman Vincent Peale, the American writer of inspirational books, is still adding to his best-sellers and lecturing worldwide and he, too, is over ninety. Sir Vivian Fuchs, the famous explorer, recently remarried at the age of 83. 'I am too lively to be old,' he is reported to have said.

Not all inspiring older people are famous: my fascinating grandmother-in-law lived busily by herself in a cold old farmhouse until she was 99, still insisting on baking cakes for my husband. I have older friends (congratulations to Zeana, Jean and Stella) who look good, dress well and live with great *joie de vivre*, for me to copy. I am sure we can all point to 'youthful' octogenarians, and 'old' forty-somethings. There are many older slim, fit, interesting and interested people in this world, but we need to look for them.

In horse-racing, the handicapper penalises the horses that he thinks can win easily, by giving them a handicap. That handicap is extra weight to carry. Extra weight is always a handicap, whether for fit racehorses, or for people. This particularly applies to people growing older, as the body may lose some of its flexibility and efficiency, unless we counteract it with how we eat and exercise.

Someone once said that 'age is not toxic'. That is, bodies are ruined by misuse and disuse rather than by the ravages of time. Over 80 per cent of wrinkles are caused by the sun, not by age. The suppleness of someone who is sixty-something can be improved by a suitable exercise programme as much as that of a twenty-something stripling of a person. It is not uncommon for workaholic men who retire to lie down and die, because they have lost their will to live. They have thought old, useless, hopeless thoughts, and so have acted old and hopeless – and died.

You can keep full of life at any age. It's not your age that matters, it's your attitudes; how you *think*, and act.

## COUNTERACT WITH THINK SLIM
- Think Slim: Age is irrelevant.
- If you think of yourself as old, you will act old – and probably think yourself into an early grave.
- Don't think old thoughts. Don't think helpless and hopeless. Don't misuse your body. And, if you don't want to lose it, use it.

## TOO TIRED!
'I'm just too tired to exercise,' moans Della.

'I'm too tired at the end of a long day to even think straight,' adds Abigail.

They are not the only ones. Doctors' waiting-rooms are populated with people complaining about the tiredness they are afflicted with. Yet, in the majority of cases, there is no physical illness causing that fatigue. Doctors are willing to check for physical problems, and it's a wise precaution to first visit your doctor for advice. Then think about the other causes of tiredness. It may be caused by a variety of factors.

### 1 POOR NUTRITION
Dieting unwisely can mean starving your body of the fuel it needs to give you energy. Certainly, you could lose weight on 850 calories of boiled eggs each day (and some people, foolishly, try to do so) but you'd be suffering from a form of malnutrition, which would make you feel tired. The eating programme in this book emphasises fitness as well as slimness, and suggests eating a variety of foods that *energise* as well as help you slim.

Also, you are requested to take a multi-vitamin/mineral tablet to ensure that you are getting enough of those vital bits that our body needs. A study from the Canadian Institute of Stress reported in 1989 by one of its directors Dr Richard Earle, showed that for reducing the debilitating effects of stress and for increasing vitality, good nutrition when accompanied by a daily multi-vitamin/mineral tablet was significantly more effective than relying on good nutrition alone. The quality of much of our food is variable, but you can rely on a good supplement (such as Boots' *Plurivite*).

**Caffeine – friend or foe?** Caffeine can be so much a hidden part of our everyday life that we never consider whether it's a real friend or a foe to our body. Caffeine is present in regular coffee, in tea and in colas. People reach for a coffee to 'keep them awake' and it works – briefly. But caffeine jump-starts the nervous system and is an artificial stressor on the body. Later, energy levels soon dive low in reaction, and another shot of caffeine is needed. Larger amounts cause irritability, and irritability/lethargy/headache withdrawal symptoms can occur if your next shot is not readily available. So, try de-caffeinated coffee, tea and cola. Do I hear, 'But I don't like it'? If you don't like one brand of de-caffeinated, try another, for there is great variety in brands and taste now available. Life is difficult and tiring enough without adding to the stresses on our body and brain with caffeine. So help yourself, with de-caffeinateds.

**Too much alcohol** can also cause tiredness, even if you don't experience a full-blown hangover. A caller recently asked advice of a radio doctor about 'the morning after' lethargy he suffers, even after only a couple of alcoholic drinks. How could he avoid it? You guessed! If alcohol tires you (and it does all of us) and you don't want to be tired, choose not to have the alcohol. You may suffer from tiredness even drinking less than the recommended 'limits', 21 units per week for men and 14 for women. (If you wish to read more about alcohol, the recommended 'limits' and its calories, refer to pages 65 and 191–2).

**Too little . . .** Maybe too little of other fluids is making you tired. Doctors advise that the body needs at least 3 pints (1.7 litres, about 9 mugs) per day to function at its best. It doesn't matter whether you 'feel' thirsty or not, drink more than you 'feel' you need. You can then 'shop and shop and never drop', or do more of whatever you want, to use up your energy.

## COUNTERACT WITH THINK SLIM
- Eat mostly high-energy foods – those low in fat and sugar, and high in fibre and complex carbohydrates, as recommended in the eating programme later in this book.
- Take a multi-vitamin/mineral tablet daily. Every day. (But do not exceed the dosage stated on the packaging.) Recommended: Boots' *Plurivite*.
- Avoid too much alcohol. Check your intake against recommended limits (page 65) and also notice how you feel the morning after alcohol.
- Make sure you have enough low-calorie fluids; at least 3 pints/1.7 litres (about 9 mugs) each day.
- Avoid caffeine. Buy de-caffeinated coffee, tea and colas.

## 2 DO-IT-ALL
If you are already eating and drinking for energy, but are still tired,

maybe you are simply suffering from trying to Do-It-All. You are trying to be Mr/Mrs/Ms Superperson, coping beautifully with everything *and* the kitchen sink; high-flying in the boardroom, multiply-orgasmic in the bedroom; perfecting the parenting process; rag-rolling the walls, organically producing the greens; hostessing elegant dinner parties for a dozen; fund-raising for charities, saving elephants and whales; caring for dependent relatives, love-torn friends, tempestuous teenagers, and birds with broken wings; dressing to impress while keeping up with the latest fashion; aerobically dancing or dauntlessly jogging. You're tired. You're surprised?

## COUNTERACT WITH THINK SLIM

- Stop trying to Do-It-All. Forget Puritanical work ethics that drive you ever harder, faster, tired-er. You have a right to live in a civilised way, and you don't have to earn that right by your performance.
- Accept that you do not have to be perfect. Perfection is for bone china, not for people. Refer again, and again, to the part in this book 'Oughta be . . . perfick' in the Negative Wizards In Our Culture section (page 62). If you are trying to be 'Mrs Goodwife', also refer repeatedly to the 'Being Mrs Goodwife' Negative Wizard section on page 87.
- After renouncing perfectionism, decide what is really important to *you*, and restrict your activities to those things. Don't try to do or be what *other* people want of you (beyond a reasonable consideration for them).
- Learn to say 'No' to others when appropriate and don't wallow in guilt about it. Being assertive in this way is showing as much respect for yourself as for others. You deserve equal respect; accept and insist on it.
- Pace yourself during your busy day, by taking short breaks. Go for a short walk, listen to a relaxing cassette, sit in your car/bathroom/garden/attic, quietly by yourself, day-dreaming positively or relaxing; do some gentle stretches, or gently shake your body out of its stiffness. Allow yourself this 'recovery time' and 'gather yourself', and you will be less tired.

## 3 NOT RAT-RACING BUT STILL TIRED?
Maybe you are doing emotional overtime, and your body is feeling the strain.

Are you worried? Depressed? Anxious? Tense? Frustrated? Angry? All of these emotions can drain you of energy. Obviously, we all suffer from some of these emotions some of the time, but if any or all of them are your regular companions, no wonder you feel fatigued.

If you want to find the answer to your tiredness, try asking yourself some questions:

'Exactly which emotions am I feeling?' (Worry? depression? anxiety?

tension? frustration? anger?)

'*Why* am I feeling them? What is it in my life or in myself that is giving rise to these feelings?'

'What is it that I'm tired of?' Answer yourself with the words 'I'm tired of . . .'

After identifying the problem(s), seek answers. There is a solution to every problem. Be a problem-solver. The solution may not be easy or immediate, but there is a solution if you will look for it.

If there is really NO solution, you are not facing a problem, you are facing a fact of life – something which just cannot be changed. That means you need to accept it. For example, if you are up-tight because you hate your large feet, this is not a problem – it's a fact of life. You then have a choice: you can accept this fact of having big feet, realistically knowing that this is no catastrophe and that you are not judgeable as a person on the size of your feet, and that while you don't like your large feet there are others in this world who have no feet; you can get involved in interesting things in life so that you turn your mind away from this issue.

Or, if you are tense because your only child is emigrating, this too is a fact of life. Your children have the right to live their own lives (and make their own mistakes), just as you have. Yes, it would be nicer if she/ he were nearby, but it is his/her decision, not yours. So, it is not a problem, it's a fact of life. Accommodate it. Make plans to write and visit, keep your relationship joyful; make new plans for your own life and leisure time.

'I've such a difficult son. He's 22, and I don't know what I'm going to do with him,' agonises Helen.

Helen cannot 'do' anything 'with' a grown-up son, or daughter. Relax, stand back, give advice gently if asked for, and be ready to help pick up the pieces later if need be. Yes, it's hard. Being a parent is hard sometimes. But your son and your relationship and your slimming are more likely to survive intact if you accept this advice. Your alternative choice is to continue awfulising over your 'problem' and making yourself tense and miserable about it. And comfort-eating yourself fatter. Then you'll have an extra problem.

If you can see a way forward through your problem, even though no answer is immediate, you will begin to feel better if you make some first moves. If you hate your job, start re-training or look for another position; if your relationship isn't rewarding, consider it, and confront the problems, with advice or counselling if needed. Don't play the 'yes but' game, where you counter 'yes, but . . .' to every possibility. It's your life, the only one you've got. It's your choice whether you stay stuck, emotionally drained, tired and overweight as you are, or whether you do something positive to change things for the better and enjoy your life.

Don't think that I am unsympathetic to how difficult it can be to change things, but I am more optimistic about the ability of every one of us to achieve changes if we will try. Sympathy may be comforting but it can't move mountains. Efforts, one small step at a time, can do so. Efforts can even move mountains of weight – your unwanted weight.

## COUNTERACT WITH THINK SLIM
- Ask yourself questions:
    'Which emotions am I feeling?'
    'Why am I feeling them?'
    'What is it that I'm tired of?'
- Seek answers. Answer yourself with 'I'm tired of . . .' Look for a solution.
- If you need advice or counselling, get it. (You could ask your doctor where to find advice, for emotional tiredness is his business as much as is disease-tiredness. Or ask at your local library for group support or self-help books. Also, checkout the Useful Addresses and Further Reading sections in this book.)

## 4 A FINAL MISCELLANY
**Boredom** makes you tired. Get yourself interested in something new. Try a few things you've never tried, including some you think you may not like. You could surprise yourself.

**Smoking** is often thought of as a stress-reliever, but it is a stress-maker for your body. It puts up your blood pressure and your pulse rate as well as damaging your lungs and increasing your risks of heart disease and of cervical cancer in women. The fact that you feel less-stressed after a cigarette shows the power of your mind; you have de-stressed yourself by thinking you will feel better; it would work if you used any other comfort-system you believed in. I use a black de-caffeinated coffee to de-stress myself rather than a cigarette. It has no physical power to relax me, but my mind and the habit has the required effect. If you smoke, you would do better to quit; get professional help if you wish. In Britain, refer to the telephone directory, or library, for your local Health Education Department.

**Pain** gobbles up your energy. If you are suffering from physical pain from any ailment, seek advice to minimise it. Maybe try alternative therapies such as hypno-therapy, acupuncture or homeopathy.

**Excess weight** drags down your energy and leaves you lethargic, listless and too tired to enjoy life. Life in the fat lane is a tiring and tired life. So, every night as you go to sleep, resolve to tackle that weight/tiredness problem every day, by persevering with your slimming and your new, better ways of eating and thinking. *Every* successful slimmer is always delighted with how much more energy she/he has compared to when overweight.
   'I never knew I could have so much energy!' marvels Carolann, with a grin as large as her hips are slim.

## COUNTERACT WITH THINK SLIM

A final few words for all tirednesses, however caused:

- Don't think tired thoughts. If you continually repeat to yourself, even almost subconsciously, 'Oh, I am tired,' you can actually increase your tiredness. Instead, repeat to yourself/make a Think Slim Prompt Card:

> I don't think tired thoughts

- Exercise actually increases energy levels, not drains them. Try a good 20–30 minutes aerobic workout at a class, or cycle, or swim/walk hard, and you will be amazed that you have more vitality after it than you did minutes before you started. Wise exercise shakes off stress and produces natural anti-depressant hormones. A study at the University of California showed that a group of volunteers who took exercise for tiredness had more energy, measured two hours later, than the group who were given a high-calorie sugar snack. Refer to Step Seven 'Move Yourself', page 199, for information about how to exercise.

If ever I mutter 'I do feel tired' my husband retorts: 'Well, you know what to do. On yer bike!'

And he's right; it works. Wake up with wise exercise.

## FEAR OF SUCCESS

'The weight's dropping off you!' Cheryl had commented, admiringly. The next morning, Sallie checked her diminishing figure in the mirror and immediately smiled in satisfaction. Then, from underneath, a little thought erupted: 'I have done really, really well . . . perhaps too well . . .'

Suddenly, Sallie felt a little uncomfortable. She wasn't at all clear about how she felt, or what she had meant by that thought, but she didn't stop to consider it; she switched her thoughts to getting ready for work, and off she went as usual.

That evening Sallie found herself with one of those Urges – the dreadful urge to eat. Before you could say size 12, she had binged a square of cheese, a pack of cheese biscuits, another cheese chunk, a large sherry and the last of the apple pie and thick cream that she had avoided all day.

Sallie had no idea why she had her Urge. But she could have stopped to consider whether the excellence of her weight losses had frightened her into sabotaging her slimming.

Implausible? No, for fear of success can confound many a slimmer – not only about slimming, but also about their whole life.

Are such slimmers crazy? No, they are coping. Coping with a fear, in the only way that they know how. Not a good way to cope, but coping nevertheless. Certainly not crazy.

Why is it that we can be afraid of success? For some of us, maybe success is something we are just not used to, and so we feel uncomfortable with it. Sallie, at school, had always been a middle-of-the-road achiever, passing her exams but never the top of the class.

'That was OK by me,' she explained. 'Nobody liked the top girls anyway.'

So, Sallie felt comfortable being just 'fairly successful', and subconsciously, she continued this pattern.

Other people have learned to be comfortable as failures. That's what they have been used to, and that is how they see themselves. 'That's the way I am,' they think, so that's how they stay, keeping themselves in line with the self-image they have of themselves, so as to feel comfortable. To many people, change can be unsettling and disturbing.

Some people dread being the centre of attention. When Josie had reached the weight she wanted, she wore a new leotard and tights and looked absolutely fabulous. But she drew me aside anxiously and whispered:

'You won't ask me to come out to the front, will you? I couldn't bear it!'

How sad that we 'can't bear' to receive the public praise to which we are entitled when we succeed.

Then again, most of us want to be liked. People, generally, are brought up to seek popularity. Women, in particular, are trained to get men to like them so that they can 'win' the best husband they can – and 'best' usually means 'richest'. Men can accept success better because their worldly success usually brings them money, and this fulfils the 'breadwinner' role that they are trained into – and then their egos are rewarded by the many women who fawn around them.

However, people who are successful run the risk of being unpopular, the target of others' envy. In the USA, success is more admired socially and more acceptable than in Britain, where success is played for, then played down. It is symptomatic of this attitude that British owners of desirable motor cars often find their cars' paintwork desecrated by enviers.

For some 'successful' slimmers, it may be that it is simply too difficult to cope with the envy spitting out from those who are less successful.

'She makes me sick!' has been the (joking?) overheard comment of many a slimmer who watches someone else lose weight in a way that she or he hasn't managed. When I hear that sort of comment I always challenge it, but maybe, often, it is a hidden thought, unchallenged, divisive, and destructive to both the thinker and its victim. For, the 'successful' one is all too uncomfortably aware of envy, whether it is spoken or unspoken. It may seem easier to slow down the success-rate or even regain weight than face such envy.

A distance can come between two friends who slim together, when one is more successful than the other. Sometimes, I've suspected that the 'successful' friend has sabotaged her own success to preserve the friendship. What unhelpful games we play! If a friend cannot accept your successful and slimline self, don't be afraid. Muster up your courage. If the envy of others loses you 'friends', their friendship wasn't worth much anyway. You can always make new friends, preferably slim-fit ones with whom you have interests in common.

Begin to think that it's OK to be successful. There can be nothing wrong with having success and enjoying it if you've earned it – and if you've slimmed, you've earned it.

Given the culture that we are brought up in it's not surprising to find envy sneakily creeping into your thoughts. But, once you are aware of it, you can put that envy to good use. For what you are envious of, you want. When you are envious of another's slim-success, simply let it strengthen your motivation. Stop the inglorious envy-thoughts and replace them by Think Slim: 'Yes, that's what I want, and if she can do it – so can I.'

The good news is that slimness is a target that is achievable by *everyone*; unlike a degree in Physics, or a career as a prima ballerina or racing jockey, or to be taller, or to change your eye colour.

## COUNTERACT WITH THINK SLIM
- Try to decipher your deep fears of success – exactly what are you afraid of? Envy? Unpopularity? Losing your friends? More expectations of you?
- Make Think Slim cards, and repeat the Think Slim thoughts often: It's OK to be successful. I accept and enjoy my successes.
- If you feel pangs of envy when you see other successful slimmers, use the envy to strengthen your motivation. Repeat Think Slim: If he/she can do it, so can I.
- Talk to other successful slimmers that you envy; you may find your envy disappear as you get to like them as real people. Ask for tips and ideas about improving your slimming strategies (but don't play the 'yes, but' game of making excuses as to why their tips won't work for you).

## FEAR – OF SEXUALITY
Fear of sexuality is often considered to be a 'women's problem' but men can be plagued by fears too, although they may less-readily admit to them because of the 'real male ever-ready-ever-confident' role that is foisted upon them by our culture.

Fears connected to sexuality can undermine slimming for both men and women. Women generally head for the biscuits, and men to the boozer. The problems of male and female generally differ, but both deserve attention, and shall be referred to separately as far as possible. However, the problems inevitably intertwine, as do our lives, so it can be helpful to both men and women to read all of this section.

It is not my intention to sit in judgement on one self-righteous side in some battle of the sexes, nor to totally blame one sex for the troubles of the other. My view of life is 'equalist': that is, that both men and women should be regarded as having equal rights, but, as well, both having equal responsibilities (to respect the other). All exploitation is wrong, whether by male or female. That means that women should not exploit men as money objects, just as men should not exploit women as sex objects. This equalist view is not always too popular with those women who want to have their rights and eschew their responsibilities. But being self-empowered means being responsible, and that may be harder work than playing dependent. The good news is that the price is worth it for the pay-off in feeling good about yourself and living your own life. Building your own sandcastles may be tough, but it's more fun.

Nor is it helpful to get into a power game of 'it's worse for we women than you men'. Life's too short to waste time playing gender war-games. We need to seek solutions for all sufferers.

Philosophy digested (at least that's calorie-free), we can consider the issues about fear of sexuality that can sabotage slimming, firstly, for women.

'One good thing about being fat is that I don't have to worry about men,' explained Coral. 'They never notice me; if I get slim I'll have all that hassle . . .'

Generally, society gives out the message that to be a woman who is fat is to be asexual; and, in reality, fat women are often sexually invisible to most men. But a slim woman is expected to be a sexual one, and is likely to be approached (or 'hassled'?) by men. Some women fear this attention, are uneasy about coping with it, and are uncomfortable with their own sexuality. Their fat obliterates their outward signs of sexuality, and so they feel safer.

Is Fat A Feminist Issue? Susie Orbach, in her book about compulsive eating, *Fat Is a Feminist Issue*, pointed out that for some women, staying fat has a purpose, albeit an unconscious one. Orbach argues that being fat is an unconscious female rebellion against becoming the sex image that male domination decrees she should be; her fat is her effort to break free from the sexual stereotype forced upon her.

Susie Orbach suggests that the fat is speaking for the woman, silently swearing: 'Screw You – take me as I am.' The fat does the job of repulsing men in a way that the woman does not feel powerful enough to do herself; she does not feel entitled to say no, so her fat says it for her.

For some women, maybe this is so. The problem with the argument is that because Orbach declares it an unconscious process, no one is able to refute it. It cannot be proved, but nor can it be disproved. If I say there is no evidence, it can be argued that that is because the unconscious mind is not available to us for evidence. I remember being overweight in those seventies-Orbach-days, and trying to search my psyche for this underlying unconscious desire to be fat to avoid being a sex object. All

I can say is that the theory didn't seem to fit me, and that my yo-yo fat-slim syndrome was defeated not by any analysis of my dreams and resolving some subconscious sexual anxieties, but by re-educating my thinking, my habits and my eating. However, Orbach did do something valuable, in that she directed our attention to the connection between our lives as women and our attitudes to eating.

For it may not be so much that 'the Fat' has a purpose, as that some women have difficulties in dealing with their sexuality and reconciling it with society's demands, and it is this ever-present dilemma and pressures that lead women to over-eat in order to cope. Such fears may present themselves as a vague free-floating anxiousness upon which such women are unable to pin a cause. They may not know what is wrong; they don't know whom to ask for help, or even what questions to ask; they don't know how to cope. So they cope the only way they have learned to cope with anxiety, stress or tension – they eat. The fat is the by-product of the eat-to-cope style.

It is hardly surprising that many women have difficulty dealing with their sexuality. Our society, which is ostensibly liberated and permissive, is in reality in a state of confusion and chaos about its sexual attitudes and mores, particularly those relating to women. Women are weighed down with dictums that give totally opposing and irreconcilable messages: 'Be the first woman he's ever had, but be uninhibited. Be a sex kitten. Be a Virgin Mary (maybe named after her). Be prepared to take off all your clothes, but only in the best possible taste. Be a saintly, servile, Mother. Be a prostitute, but be ostracised from acceptable society. Be 'topless' but be taunted and compared. Be a decent fragrant wife but be a whore when he wants it. Be assaulted and raped but be quiet or the neighbours will hear or the judge will accuse you of askin' for it.

There's always a 'Catch 69'. If a woman obeys and becomes sexually available she may be insulted as a 'slag'; if she obeys the opposing commandment, waiting as a 'nice girl' with legs demurely crossed, she may be dismissed as a 'tight bitch'.

Men, too, have not escaped the confusion of these messages; they have inherited the conflicting ideas about women that are related above. They can't reconcile the notions either. So, we read of an arrested kerb crawler who admitted: 'I suppose I'm sexually repressed'; he couldn't relax with his 'nice' wife to enjoy the sexual relationship he sought. Hardly surprising in a society where Judges still make pronouncements about 'unnatural practices' when they mean oral sex. A recent survey indicated over 60 per cent of men were dissatisfied with their sex lives. It's my guess that if their partners were interviewed, at least as many (if not more) would be expressing a similar lack of satisfaction. We tell surveys; we don't tell our partners.

How does society weigh down women and men in these ways? 'They fuck you up, your Mum and Dad.' First, although we are all born as naturally sexual beings, from early childhood we soon learn to feel guilty and anxious about sexuality. Parents generally stay resoundingly silent on the subject and do not even reveal the names of our sexual bits and pieces. Both boy- and girl-children, daring to touch their own genitals in natural exploration, are very likely to be reprimanded. Even some tampons are designed to remind us that Ladies don't touch, and have an applicator so as to avoid a woman's finger coming into contact with her vagina (yet she must be a sex kitten when he wants it).

Second, while schools teach us how to do long division, to parrot 'Je m'appelle', and to light bunsen burners, they fail to offer any planned and adequate sex education.

Also, we are the inheritors of churches' preaching that sexuality is solely for the procreation of children. Male masturbation was therefore a sin (because it spilled the seed that could have produced a child). Female masturbation was apparently so inconceivable it was not mentioned; although, in the 19th century, male doctors regarded it as causing madness in women, so that women showing signs of psychiatric disturbance were often circumcised (that is, the clitoris and surrounding area were mutilated).

Up to the 1960s, lack of good birth control meant that sexual intercourse often led to pregnancy after tiring pregnancy. Many women preferred a 'good' husband – one who didn't bother them much.

As children inherited their father's wealth, and fathers did not relish a bastard child being foisted on them, women were not encouraged to enjoy sex in case they indulged elsewhere. Also, women were kept in their sexual place (horizontal under their dominant husbands) by being insulted as 'tarts/slags/whores' if they chose many partners (while men doing the same were praised as Don Juans and studs).

Society changed with the waning influence of the churches, the pill and permissive attitudes prompted by the media of the swinging sixties. But even in the sixties (and ever since) swinging women may still be called slags, or by new names such as 'old dog'.

Recently, at a sex-education course for professionals that I was leading, a man, having already described himself as being sexually liberated by the sixties, later spoke of some women at a social function, waiting to be 'picked up – just like a cow market'. When these words were challenged, he apologised: 'I should have said cattle market.' He didn't even understand what the challenge to his words was about. This 'liberated' male was still displaying a dubious sort of liberation for him, but not for her.

Romantic pap rules pop songs and teenage magazines, and encourages emotions to ruin rational thought and realistic expectations. There remains sexual angst and anxiety, uncertainty and ignorance; and over 180,000 abortions last year in Britain alone to prove it. For people change less quickly than media fashions, and we inheritors of the old thought-habits, guilts and anxieties, flounder and suffer. Many of us eat.

For young men growing up, society has had one consistent and straightforward message about sex – get it.

It's crude, uncaring (and therefore abhorrent). The pressures are different from those on women, but the pressures, to compete, conquer and score, are real and debilitating. The fear of rejection must be overcome, time and time again, while it is the woman who has the power and pleasure of giving that first yea or nay. Some of those pressures can at least be dealt with, partly, by pretending (to have won, vanquished and scored). But there are no friendly shoulders to confide fears to, at the bar or the rugby club. Men's fears and anxieties are often washed away with calorie-laden alcohol, or maybe bigger portions on their plates. Their slimming is sabotaged.

Another Men Only problem is the outward and visible sign of their manhood; the comparison game in the boys' changing rooms, the fears primed by 'is-it-big-enough?' jokes. (A fear being prompted recently even in one of the new men's magazines.) Further, he is expected to give a Command Performance: to be a self-starter and ever-ready. Anything less and he is a wimp. (That's another dreadful, destructive four-letter word.) His fears about Can't Get It Up are as bad as the fears about Can't Get It. Both stem from our culture's definition of sex (sex = sexual intercourse), and the roles that have emerged, without rational thought, and been inflicted upon men and women. (Life as a Mills and Bornographic Script.)

It's time for a massive, rational re-think and a major re-education.

Another male fear, that he might lose his sexual partner, may lead HIM to sabotaging HER slimming.

Peter appeared to be the tall, dark, handsome officer and gentleman type of man on whose arm you might expect some stunning model-girl. But she-by-his-side was, frankly, very fat and frumpy. He confided in me: 'At least, I can be sure she won't leave me for another man, because no one will fancy her.' How sad that his fears of being sexually and emotionally abandoned had pressed him into choosing a partner for such a negative reason. How sad that she would be encouraged to remain fat and frumpy to assuage his fears, and sad that she would never know why he liked her fat. (No, I didn't tell her. His was a confidence. Interestingly, their relationship broke up after about ten months. She was still fat and frumpy.)

Other men feel threatened for a similar reason when their partners are seen to be slimming successfully. He sees 'his' woman becoming more attractive, more confident, more assertive, more popular, and he becomes more afraid. Both men and women have to live with the threat of abandonment; we can minimise that fear by making real efforts to keep our relationships alive and interesting. The slimming woman can take time and thought to reassure her man that she still values him, and that they can enjoy her slimmer world much better, together.

But neither partner should expect 'the magic' to magically remain.

'The magic's not there any more,' complained David. David is living in fantasyland. Fantasies may be OK, but not when we begin to believe in them. David, and the rest of us, need to create our own magic, and re-create it continuously. 'Making it' involves us making it happen. Loving relationships only stay that way if we continue to behave lovingly. And if our partner is slipping into comfortable slippers and inconsiderate habits, we need to tell him/her, gently, that we want something better.

Also, we need to keep the threat of abandonment in proportion. If the worst happened, how 'worst' would it really be? Yes, we can make it 'worst'; people can be good at creating a tragic drama out of a crisis. (Some women prefer to play Hedda Gabler than Pollyanna. Pollyanna had a nicer time.) More positively, we could decide that we would cope. First, we would hurt, and cry and mourn and that would be right; then we would cope. Clarissa, one year after her own crisis, rang me to say delightedly: 'You were right. I haven't been so happy for years.'

Far from there being only one Mr/Ms Right out there, there are literally millions of other men and women also looking for relationships. We can cope, recover, survive and be happy again, if we will only be active about finding someone, and fussy that we choose someone who is suitable rather than merely convenient or the fulfilment of some fairytale fantasy.

Alternatively, it's OK to be single. It's not compulsory to be a twosome. The thought of abandonment is easier to live with, and less likely to rule our actions, when we rationally consider it happening, and ourselves surviving.

**'No sex please, it's 9 to 5'**: Women of the 1990s are often not just working women but ambitious women on the way up. For some of them, there is another fear connected to slimness and sexuality. They want to avoid being seen as a sex symbol in the workplace because they may not be taken seriously as career women. This is another difficult role, as they are still faced with the injunction to turn into sex kittens at the stroke of five.

Such women may deal with the pressures of this schizophrenic-style dual role by eating. Or, they may wish to de-sexualise their appearance and, as suggested by Susie Orbach, fatten themselves into sexual neutrality for the boardroom.

How can all these pressures be alleviated, apart from by comfort-eating?

There is a way out, apart from eating cake. On a societal level, in our schools we need good quality sex education that will teach boys and girls to accept their sexuality as natural rather than shameful, to be equally caring of each other and equally responsible; to believe that people are precious beings, born to relate to each other, not convenient objects to be carelessly used, abused and cast aside by self-centred selves.

In our media we need responsible thinkers who will eschew profit for principles. Fat chance! Instead, we will probably need tighter regulation of sexual exploitation and violence, and the courage to demand it.

Individual women and men need some re-education, which can start here. The dilemmas that society heaps upon women and men cannot easily be resolved, but they can first be confronted and then their irrationality and chaos rejected.

In another strand of my professional life, I teach sex education to various groups of people (including sex offenders). I find myself consulted by 1990s people with these very problems. The death threat of AIDS adds to their concerns. The approach I suggest is below.

## COUNTERACT WITH THINK SLIM
**Both men and women:**
- Think through the sexual messages you have received, and still receive, through your life. What were they? Were there many negative ones, such as that sex is shameful, or that women have less sexual rights than men?
- Recognise that conflicting demands are impossible; think which to dismiss.
- Read more about sexuality (refer to the Further Reading list, page 276); think and talk more.
- Consider whether any fear of sexuality is sabotaging your slimming efforts, and in what way.
- Talk to friends and partners about sexuality in general, and talk to your partner about your relationship in particular. Are you both satisfied with your sexual relationship at present; if not, why not?
- Get counselling help if you have problems you cannot easily resolve. Contact your local branch of Relate (formerly the Marriage Guidance Council), or consult a qualified private counsellor.

**Women:**
- Tell him if you have that common dilemma – that you know that if you have sex you may be called a slag; that if you don't, you may be called a neurotic. Open up a discussion, and then do what *you* choose to do. It's not only your life, it's *your* sexuality.

**Finally:**
- Accepting your sexuality and expressing it (responsibly, while respecting yourself and your partner) can add immeasurably to your enjoyment in life. And, it's far more compatible with a slim-fit lifestyle than is swallowing your feelings with a box of Belgian chocolates or a crate of beer.

## *FEAR – FROM SEXUAL ABUSE OR ATTACK*
For some women, fear of sexuality unfortunately has traumatic roots, because they have been sexually abused, attacked or raped. They may

now recoil from sexual encounters, and over-eat to keep their fatness as an unconscious attempt to remain sexually invisible to men at large.

One rape-survivor relates: 'I wanted to be unattractive; fat helped me. I didn't wear make up or bother with my appearance at all.'

Unfortunately, being overweight is little defence against abuse or attack; sex offenders often attack any female who happens to be geographically convenient and is seen as a relatively 'easy' target to intimidate or overpower.

In the USA, there is increasing awareness of 'date-rape'. That is where a woman has accepted a date with a man who later refuses to take her 'no' as an answer to his sexual advances, and rapes her. Women suffering such an experience often don't report the man to the police, yet they may be shattered by the experience.

They too may see their fatness as protecting them from further attack. Alternatively, their continuing failure at slimming is due to the extra eating they do, in an attempt to comfort themselves and quieten their anxiety, tension, guilt or horror.

Sometimes sexual abuse may have been suffered a long time ago, when the slimmer was a child. Adult slimmers may not connect their failure to slim with that experience. Men, as well as women, may be abused as children. Both sexes may, as adults, suffer long-term anxiety or tension that seems to have no cause but results in comfort eating or binges.

One American Clinic treating eating disorders reported that 80 per cent of its clients had been sexually abused when younger.

Sometimes adults also carry a heavy burden of guilt that began in their childhood, after being abused, as if they were partly to blame. Children and adults who have been abused or attacked need to be reassured that it was not their fault, that the responsibility lies *only* with the perpetrator. Any feelings of guilt need to be swept away, and feelings of anger against the offender may need to be expressed.

If you are a parent it can be traumatic if you find that your child has been abused or attacked. You may need assistance to deal positively with your feelings rather than turn to food, and to help you best cope with the child and hishe/her feelings. (In Britain, the Kate Adams Crisis Centre would advise you. Tel: (081) 593 9428.)

## COUNTERACT WITH THINK SLIM
- Anyone who has been abused or attacked needs to seek help. If you are constantly failing at slimming and you have had abusive experiences, it is possible that you are sabotaging your slimming in an unproductive attempt to deal with your experiences. There are organisations in Britain which can be contacted for assistance (see Useful Address section, page 273). Otherwise your doctor should be able to advise you where you can obtain counselling.
- To get counselling is the wise and mature way to survive abuse or

attack. Even if it seems hard to take that first step, do so, as it won't be as bad as you may imagine because sensitive trained counsellors are available. Don't postpone your relief.

# CHECKLIST: IDENTIFY YOUR NEGATIVE WIZARDS

Now you have read and thought about many possible saboteurs that may have ruined your slimming in the past, and could have the power to spoil your efforts in the future, it is time to take action.

You are invited to put your thoughts into gear, and put pen to paper. If you wish to slim successfully, you need to do both. (If you think you can't be bothered or that you haven't got time, think again.)

**ACTION**
- Read through the following checklist, and think about all the possible saboteurs that exist for you: in Your Life, in our Culture, in Yourself.
- Identify (honestly) the ones that affect you, and tick in the boxes below.

## 1 NEGATIVE WIZARDS IN YOUR LIFE
Are there people like this in your life?

|  |  |  | Tick if it applies to you |
|---|---|---|:---:|
| 1 The Commander: | Warns, 'You shouldn't be ...' | | ☐ |
| 2 The Jailer: | She/he locks away the biscuits ... | | ☐ |
| | Or, do you even invite someone to be your 'jailer'? | | ☐ |
| 3 The Put-downer: | Puts you down: 'You're not on *another* diet!' | | ☐ |
| 4 The Spoiler: | Buys you high-cal treats. | | ☐ |
| | Tempts: 'Go on, spoil yourself!' | | ☐ |
| 5 The Smotherer: | Looks after you like a (s)motherer ... | | ☐ |
| | Over-fills you up with food, over-protects you. | | ☐ |

## 2 NEGATIVE WIZARDS IN OUR CULTURE

Are you listening to cultural messages that sabotage your slimming?
Do your thoughts begin to echo these sabotaging messages?

1 Eat, drink and be merry:　'If you want to be merry you must eat and drink!'　□

2 Instantism:　Want it Now! Instant results! Instant slimming!　□

3 Never too thin:　Thin is In, Thinner is even better!　□

4 Oughta-bee . . . Perfick:　You Ought to be the Perfect . . . mum, wife, highflyer, husband, sex symbol, lover, slimmer . . .　□

5 The Super-slimmer syndrome:　Do it quicker, with bigger weight losses, and be a Super-slimmer.　□

6 Excess-ism:　More, more, more! Eat more! Drink more! He/she who eats and drinks Most is Best!　□

## 3 NEGATIVE WIZARDS IN YOURSELF

Are *you* harbouring thoughts that sabotage your slimming?
Do you recognise any of these saboteurs within yourself, coming from your own thoughts — thoughts that have become a habit?

1 The Wooden Leg Syndrome:　'You can't expect me to slim, I've got . . .'　□

2 Living in Never Never Land:　'I'll Never lose all this weight.'　□

'I'll Never reach . . . ; I'll Never . . .'　□

3 Not in the Mood:　'I'm just not in the mood!' 'I'll wait till . . .'　□

4 The Ostrich Position:　'I don't think I'll like it!'　□

5 'I Should Be So Lucky':　'She's lucky . . .'　□

6 Yes, But-er:　'Yes but'. (To all suggestions: 'yes, I would, but I can't because . . .')　□

7 The Wisher:　'I wish I was slim.' 'I wish I could lose weight like she does.' 'I wish . . .'　□

| | | |
|---|---|---|
| 8 Poor Me!: | 'I feel so deprived.' 'I can't have . . .' | ☐ |
| 9 The Cinders Syndrome: | Waiting – for a fairy godmother, magic or a Miracle. | ☐ |
| 10 Not Enough Time: | 'I've Not Enough Time!' To plan, prepare, cook, exercise, slim . . . | ☐ |
| 11 The Urge: | 'Then I get this dreadful Urge (to eat).' | ☐ |
| | 'Only to cheer myself up.' | ☐ |
| 12 Not Fair!: | 'It's not fair . . . she can eat anything.' | ☐ |
| 13 The Demon Imp: Impatience: | 'I want to be slim, tomorrow.' | ☐ |
| 14 The Demon Imp: Impulse: | 'OK, I'll just have . . .' | ☐ |
| 15 Being Mrs Goodwife: | 'I have to prove what a Goodwife I am . . .' | ☐ |
| 16 The Secret Eater: | 'No one sees me over-eat. If no-one sees me, it won't count.' | ☐ |
| 17 That Li'l Bit: | 'That Li'l Bit won't hurt (to eat).' | ☐ |
| 18 Fat Habits: | 'I always have a . . .' | ☐ |
| 19 The Nega-thinker: | 'It's so depressing, slimming.' 'I can't be bothered to . . .' | ☐ |
| 20 Not At My Age: | 'I'm too old to bother . . .' | ☐ |
| 21 Too Tired!: | 'I'm too tired to exercise, to change . . . even to think.' | ☐ |
| 22 Fear – of Success: | 'Don't feel comfortable as a success.' | ☐ |
| 23 Fear – of Sexuality: | 'Don't feel comfortable seen as a sexual person.' | ☐ |
| 24 Fear – from Sexual Abuse or Attack: | 'Bad sexual experiences lead me to avoid sexual encounters.' | ☐ |

Any other personal sabotaging thoughts?
Think, and write in for yourself:

......................................................................................................................

......................................................................................................................

## MORE ACTION
- Re-read the Negative Wizard Section(s) that apply to you so that you are totally aware of what you need to counteract.
- Then read the following section about how to respond, and begin to think about your plans to get rid of the saboteurs.

## RESPONDING TO NEGATIVE WIZARDS
Don't lie back and think of England. Whether the Sabotage is from other people, from our cultural messages (such as adverts) or from within yourself, you need an *active* and *positive* response.

Following are suggestions for responding to saboteurs, and they apply even if you are responding to your own sabotaging thoughts. You need to talk back to yourself. (Nobody will take you away for it – not as long as you talk sense!)
- You need to be prepared for negative encounters of any kind, and be ready with an answer.
- It is better to respond to Negative Wizards with an answer, rather than to ignore them. This is because of two factors:

   By actively answering, you empower yourself: you assert your own self and increase your overall confidence.

   By repeating the Think Slim principles that you believe in (either aloud to others, or silently to yourself), you fix them even more firmly in your thoughts.

   *Both of these factors maximise your chances of slimming success.*
- Your Think Slim answer is more useful if it is learned, ready to trip off your tongue. For example, 'I'm *not* on a diet – I'm slimming, and I can have this'.
- The answer is better if it is positive rather than being a 'cutting remark' in retaliation. Apart from allowing you to keep your friends, a positive answer reinforces your Think Slim approach, refuses to allow inappropriate guilt, and does not escalate anger. It encourages you to remain calm and sure of yourself, avoiding shattering your slimming composure.
- As time goes on, you will find it easier to create your positive Think Slim answers ad lib; but at first you need to think ahead, learn some useful phrases, and so be prepared.
- If the Negative Wizard persists, don't be drawn into an argument. Repeat your Think Slim answer, *in exactly the same words*, as often as it's needed.
- If the Negative Wizard is another person who is close to you (such as partner, mother, or best friend), choose a calm moment to explain the principles of your Think Slim approach, and say something like: 'I would really appreciate it if you would help me by encouraging me. I feel discouraged when you . . . (include what she/he says or does). I know you're trying to help, and I'm glad, but I'd like you to . . . (include the support you would like). I know I can slim with your help.'

Alternatively, read some of this book out aloud to the Negative Wizard, and discuss it together. Or, buy him/her a copy of hishe/her own! (It costs less than a big box of chocolate or a silk tie!)

- Make yourself a list of the Think Slim answers you intend to use when confronted by a Negative Wizard. (There is space below, or you can make yourself a Think Slim journal or scrap book.)
- Review your list and your Think Slim answers *often*; do not chastise yourself for occasional failures to follow your plans; just read them again, again, and again – and start yourself off again.

## YOUR CHOSEN THINK SLIM PHRASES

**Name of Negative Wizard**       **Your 'Think Slim' answers**

.................................................................................................................

.................................................................................................................

.................................................................................................................

.................................................................................................................

.................................................................................................................

.................................................................................................................

.................................................................................................................

.................................................................................................................

.................................................................................................................

.................................................................................................................

.................................................................................................................

.................................................................................................................

# MOTIVATE YOURSELF!
## Life's too short
## to live it fat!

'I wore a baggy cardi last summer all through that heat, just to hide my bulk,' began Janette, 'but nothing really hides it. Next summer, I want to be slim enough to wear anything I like.'

I remember a summer too hot, with a 'me' who was too fat to wear anything from my bulging wardrobe. I bought two tents in a pretty, cool, voile cotton and I wore them shapelessly, repeatedly and miserably throughout that heat. Never again, I vowed.

You are reading this book. That is outward evidence that you have an inner spark – motivation – that is driving you towards slim-fitness.

It is motivation that spurs us into action. The main motivation that spurs us to slim-fitness consists of two equally important parts.

| THINK WHY | + | THINK POSSIBLE |
|---|---|---|
| (Reasons to be slim-fit) | + | (Belief that it's possible) |

If we have reasons to be slim, but no belief that it's possible, we have despair, and we shall not take the action needed.

On the other hand, if we believe being slim is possible, but have no reason for wanting slimness, we shall not make the efforts needed to achieve it.

Slimming needs real effort, over a long period of time, so you need motivation that is strong. That spark within you needs to be fanned into a flame, burning brightly and strongly, impelling you into action to get yourself slim-fit.

Unfortunately, it is only in wonderland that Alices can find a magic bottle labelled 'Drink Me' that could provide the magic of motivation. Nor is it any use to 'wait' for motivation to burn bright. Just as when you light a fire, you need to fan the sparks into flame and have to tend it regularly to keep it burning bright, motivation needs building.

I am sure that you have learned enough already from this book to know who is responsible for the job of building up your motivation. Yes, you. It is a task that you can do successfully, because this chapter will teach you how.

You already possess that spark of motivation. Maybe you are still wondering whether or not it's worth making the effort to embark on this Think Slim programme.

# 1 STRENGTHEN YOUR MOTIVATION: 'THINK WHY' – REASONS TO BE SLIM-FIT

There is a Fat liberation movement that argues that Fat is OK; that the rest of the world is wrong to 'discriminate' against fatness. I disagree.

Fat is patently not OK. I have experienced fat and I've experienced slim and I know that Life in the Fat Lane is life in slow motion. Fat is not OK for romping on the floor with your baby or your grandchildren; not OK for fulfilling the urge to run, out of sheer exhuberance; not OK for allowing you to express any joy in a physical way; not OK for making love in any position you fancy; not OK for sliding into a Porsche, or into a racing car at an Activity Centre, or for sneaking a go on the children's swing; not OK for running with the Alsatian, or running after the Norwegian Naval Officer. Whatever you choose to enjoy, it's not so enjoyable when you're Fat. One Slimmer of the Year was heard to say, about her fat life: 'I never knew what I was missing!' She was right. A fat life is a second best, lack-lustre life. Life's too short to live it fat!

Do you agree? If so, fix these ideas firmly and repeatedly in your thoughts to fuel your motivation.

If you don't agree, I can't help you yet. Read on for inspiration, or abandon this book and stay fat, until the day you are ready to rethink.

To strengthen our motivation we need not only to have reasons to be slim, but we need to be very consciously aware of those reasons.

'I want to wear shorts and feel good!' Pat stated.

'I want to wear all those clothes that are in my wardrobe that are too tight!'

'I've always been called "That Big Blonde", admitted Karen, 'and I don't want to be That Big Blonde any more!'

'I'm going on holiday with a group of people and I'm far the fattest, and I want to surprise them by the pool.'

'I want to have sex with the light on, and not feel embarrassed about my size.'

'I want to wear my French knickers without the fat bulging through the lace!'

'I don't want my children to be embarrassed by my size on school Open Days.'

'I want to shop somewhere else instead of the Outsize Shop!'

'I want to improve my health.'

Good health is something that we may take for granted until it's gone. There are many illnesses that are related to overweight, or made worse by it: High blood pressure, Breast cancer, Gallstones, Hip problems, Knee joint problems, Varicose veins, Strokes, Heart troubles, Back ache/strain, Womb problems.

## BUILD YOUR MOTIVATION: 'THINK WHY'

- Think Slim: 'Life's Too Short To Live It Fat!'
- Think about *your* own reasons to be slim. Your reasons to be slim will be individual to you. Allow yourself some time to think about this.
- Write down as many as you can think of. (Can you find 20?) These need to be written down to give them emphasis.
- Re-read your reasons to be slim, often, and particularly if you notice that your motivation is flagging. Motivation, like vitamins, must be taken regularly for best effect.

## 2 STRENGTHEN YOUR MOTIVATION: 'THINK POSSIBLE' – BELIEVE THAT IT'S POSSIBLE

You have reasons to be slim; now you need to strengthen your belief that it is possible for you. You do this by focusing on and accepting the following fundamental beliefs about the slimming that you are about to start.

Fundamental Beliefs:

1 No matter how much weight you have to lose – it is possible for you to be slim.
2 No matter how long you have been overweight – it is possible for you to be slim.
3 No matter how many times you have failed on diets before – it is possible for you to be slim.
4 No matter how much you doubt your own present capabilities – it is possible for you to be slim.

Just pause for a moment to check your own reactions to reading those fundamental beliefs. What thoughts have you had already? Do any of those statements seem acceptable – unlikely – impossible – for you? Which statements do you believe? Are you already thinking 'No chance!' to any/some/all of them?

You need to believe all of them if you are to slim successfully. It doesn't matter if at this moment you don't accept them; but over a period of time, you need to work at accepting them as your own, building up your own confidence in them.

They are true statements, but maybe your past experiences have led you to doubt them now. However, in the past you have been trying to get slim with diets, and no one taught you how to slim by adopting a new, better lifestyle for a lifetime, with both your eating and your thinking.

Consider the statements in terms of this new approach and with the facts and some rational (not emotional) thinking. For, there is irrefutable evidence for each of those beliefs:

**1 No matter how much weight you have to lose – it is possible for you to be slim.** The laws of nature apply to everyone (even you – yes?). If you cut yourself, you bleed. If you bash yourself hard enough, you bruise. If you eat less than your unique body needs to carry on its life, you lose weight. You do not have to be an Einstein at Maths to understand this simple equation.

It might feel as if you put weight on when you stand near a Belgian chocolate, but it is not true.

There are too many people in the world – failed dieters who wish to defend themselves, and 'experts' who are too ignorant or too naïve or too 'kind' and so believe the failed dieters – who will try to convince you that slimming is 'impossible' for some people. They might be well-intentioned, but they are misguided and mistaken.

The (often slim) 'experts' believe the survey-answers given by dieters as to what and how much they eat. I know (don't you?) that people being surveyed are economical with their calorie-truth. In surveys, no one admits to buying the popular newspaper that outsells all others. Few vote the way they say that they will, in surveys. Surveys are little more than useless. When slimmers are hospitalised and supervised and their dressing gown pockets are searched, they lose weight. It *is* possible.

Sally Cline, writing in her book *Just Desserts*, of dieters who don't lose weight, is prepared to believe them when they protest their over-eating innocence, yet she accepts that anorexics and bulimics practise deception. She is trying to be kindly and understanding, but only succeeds in being naïve. It is not kind to allow people to deceive the world and kid themselves, and stay suffering, trapped in their fat. The fact is that:

The laws of nature apply to everyone.

We are overweight because we over-eat (that is, over-eat for our individual body's needs and our level of activity).

The most potent and simple evidence for this truth is that you never see a size 26 in a starving Third World country.

This belief says that it *is* possible for you to be slim. It is not claiming that it is easy. But it is *possible* – and you need to firmly believe that. Help yourself to accept this first belief by re-reading this paragraph, and repeating the evidence, often. You know it makes sense. Don't play kid-yourself games.

**2 No matter how long you have been overweight – it is possible for you to be slim.** The evidence for this belief is exactly the same as for the previous one. Nature isn't age-ist. It doesn't discriminate on the grounds of age. Yes, your ageing body can become a little more sluggish at using up its calories, but that doesn't disprove this belief. You can help your body work more efficiently, and Step 7 in this book (see page 199) explains how. But, fundamentally, nature's laws apply, however long you have been overweight. If you went to live in a starving Third World country, after being overweight for 50 years, you would still starve.

Joan is a 61-year-old Think Slimmer who has lowered her weight to a slim level that she has not been for over 30 years, before her son was born. She is not unique. Phyllis is 60-and-a-lot and has now reduced from 16 stones/102 kilos to 10 stones/63½ kilos. Chris is down to a weight lower than on the day she married, 27 years ago.

If it is possible for them, it is possible. It is therefore possible for you. Build up your belief by looking for other role models such as these, both in magazine features and around you in life. When you see such successes, stop thoughts such as: 'I bet they touched up the picture!' or 'She must be wonderful . . . I could never . . .' They are not fakes, freaks or fantastically gifted. They did it because it is possible, they found out how and they made the efforts. (You may choose not to make the efforts, and that's your choice . . . but then that's quite a different story.)

It is possible.

**3 No matter how many times you have failed on diets before – it is possible for you to be slim.** It is still possible for you to succeed this time because you are not going on yet another diet; you are learning new strategies for getting slim-fit and staying slim-fit. This time, you are learning not only about changing how you eat, but changing how you think and how you live.

You have never tried this before. This book can guide you. There is no rush; you have all the time in the world to readjust yourself and your life. You don't have to be perfect nor pressured, and if you have setbacks you can practise bouncing back rather than giving up.

Refuse to look back at your failures and allow them to haunt you.

**4 No matter how much you doubt your own present capabilities – it is possible for you to be slim.** Past failures at dieting can make you doubt your own inner capabilities. Past failures mean that present efforts can be doomed to failure because people have lost their confidence in their own capabilities. This saps their motivation.

They have, in effect, learned to be 'help-less'. Lack of hope in your *mind* – being 'hope-less' – leads to being hopeless and helpless in your *life*.

Psychologists have induced 'learned helplessness' in rats in experiments where the rats' efforts to escape from electric shocks have been randomly blocked. The rats become behaviourally hopeless and helpless, and fail to achieve their escape because of their panic or despair.

The effect of 'learned helplessness' on failed dieters may cause a similar incapacitating effect. Tension, panic, despair set in, more eating is done and another attempt at slimming is aborted. Making the next try even more likely to fail.

However, you can learn to counteract your past experiences of failure and your present thoughts of being incapable. You can rebuild your confidence and your motivation by re-thinking your views of yourself and of the power of your thoughts.

Within you, you have the power to achieve whatever you want – when you believe that you can. This is not a modern psychological theory; it is a truth recognised as long ago as a thousand years by the wise ancient Roman philosopher, Virgil, who wrote: 'they can because they think they can'.

People limit themselves and their achievements by their beliefs and their thoughts. Once it was thought that no man could run a mile in under four minutes. It was impossible, they (the nega-thinkers) declared. One man thought that it was possible, and he did it. Britain's Roger Bannister made the impossible possible when he ran a mile in 3 minutes 59.4 seconds. Since he showed it was possible, others have improved on his achievement. The New Zealander, John Walker, made it 3 minutes 49.4 seconds.

They did it because they thought they could.

It is only a thought you have to change.

## BUILD YOUR MOTIVATION: 'THINK POSSIBLE'

- If ever you doubt that slimming is somehow possible for you (or other individuals) because you are somehow unlucky or different, Think Slim: 'You never saw a size 26 in a starving Third World country.'
- What doubts, exactly, do you have about these Think Possible beliefs? Stop to check. Sit for a while, by yourself quietly, to think and bring out your doubts. Write them down if you wish. It is important to make yourself aware of your own doubts, so that you can dissolve them.

  Then consider the doubts in the light of rational thought, and the arguments presented above. Discuss your doubts with a friend you can trust to be supportive, rational and positive.
- Remind yourself regularly of the 'Four Minute Mile Story'. Keep the words 'Four Minute Mile' ready in your mind to pop out and counteract any doubt-thoughts that intrude in your mind.
- Write out Virgil's words: 'they can because they think they can'.
- Cut a large piece of card. Write on it boldly in wide felt-tip pen:

I CAN'T

Now, fold the card, vertically between the N and the ', like this

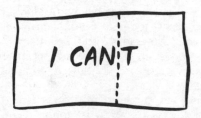

Bend right back the piece of the card that bears the T.

Your card now reads: 'I CAN'.

You can change your can't-thought to 'I can', in a similarly simple way. Keep your card, to remind you.

Catch the thought – every time those negative words 'I can't' appear in your mind – and use the Thought-stopping Technique. Say to yourself: STOP! Replace the negative thought with the positive thought: I CAN.

## MORE THINK SLIM MOTIVATORS

**Think Forward.** 'Everything in life has to be paid for,' is a realistic think saying of one of my slimmers. Absolutely right.

Many things which we need to learn in life involve a period of learning that may be somewhat painful, but is worth it, for its future gain. For example: a baby, learning to walk, tumbling down many times but scrambling up again; practising the fingering on a piano or on a typewriter; learning to drive; learning any new job; studying for exams.

The period of present pain needs to be endured. It is unrealistic to think that achievements can be made without effort. As Edison is reputed to have said: 'Genius is one per cent inspiration and 99 per cent perspiration.'

Think realistically; think forward. You can stand the present pain of changing your eating and exercising habits because you know there will be future gain – a slim-fit you, leading a more enjoyable life.

When the going gets tough, repeat the phrase 'present pain – future gain' to yourself, and persevere.

**Think rationally** about your eating and your weight: what you eat you work off – or you wear.

'Somehow I don't connect what I eat with my size,' commented Sharon. This is a 'disassociation' motivated by not wanting to accept an unpalatable truth. Start to think rationally; re-educate yourself by repeating to yourself, often, often: 'what I eat, I work off or wear.'

Don't kid yourself ('This Li'l Bit won't hurt . . .'); don't think excuses ('I had to finish off Lucy's ice cream . . .').

'I know it makes sense, but somehow I can't feel it.' Sometimes our emotional self lags behind our rational self. For slimming, we need to keep our rational self in charge of our emotional self. Your emotional self will catch up if you persist in educating it by repeating your rational reasons.

What is it that you can't emotionally convince yourself of? Confront it, rewrite the rational view and repeat it to yourself; talk to others about it; reinforce the rational. Your emotional self will catch up.

**Think Enthusiastic.** Even if you don't feel very enthusiastic, think enthusiastic thoughts. Repeat 'I'm doing fine with my slimming!' You probably are – it's only that impatient old demon imp that wants faster results, and he's got to be banished. Think enthusiasm and you'll feel it.

**Think Positive.** 'I'm on the right track,' is positive-think when you have a weight loss of half a pound/250 grammes.

Acknowledge your successes; think optimistically about your slim-fit future.

**Think-Stop the Negative.** Make your thoughts into a Negative-free Zone. Use the Thought-stopping Technique (say to yourself: STOP) and banish any Negative Wizard 'I'll never . . .' thought-dampeners.

Replace such thoughts with positive ones that begin 'I will . . . ', or use: 'I'm absolutely determined to be slim-fit'.

Repeat this thought very often. Charlotte reported that doing this made all the difference to her attitude, and results. She repeated it while walking her dog, repeating it in time, like a poem, with her footsteps. It's a good way to get yourself in the best frame of mind.

**Think Action.** None of these thoughts will be of any use unless they are followed by appropriate action.

Think Action by thinking 'I'll do it'. Then do it.

## ACTION THAT MOTIVATES

- 'Act as if . . .' Psychologists suggest that when you don't feel like doing something, ask yourself: 'What would I be doing right now if I felt motivated?' Then, simply, do whatever it is. That is, act as if you were motivated. For example: if I felt motivated I might get on my exercise bike. So, get on the bike. Simply 'act as if . . .' rather than wait for the motivation. Usually the motivation comes along when you are part way through. Whether or not it does, you still win – you'll be slimmer.
- Create a balanced lifestyle. We are 'whole' human beings who need a balanced lifestyle. All work and no play makes Jack a dull boy (it affects Jill, too), and may even have heart attack dangers. Get your life into balance. Think whether the balance is right, now. Do you need more or less of some aspects?

    Think about: your work
    your relationships, partner, family, friends
    your leisure time
    your interests/hobbies
    your relaxation time
    your holiday time.

Your slimming needs to be one aspect of a varied life.

- Create an interesting lifestyle. It's your life. If it's boring, it's you who is responsible for making it more interesting. If this is a problem area, read Step 5 Overcoming Obstacles, 'Boredom' (see page 136).
- Look around for good role models, examples of people who have succeeded in achieving the slimness that you want. Don't dismiss those who are famous, just because they are rich. Joan Collins seems a good role model to me, because she works hard to keep her looks,

and has a realistic attitude to effort and results. Yes, the rich have an advantage over you and me as they probably have less stress from an over-worked lifestyle. (Although for poor little rich girl Tina Onassis it worked against her. For when you can order any sort of delicious food at any time of the day or night by a wave of the hand and it appears almost instantaneously, your food cravings can be so easily satisfied.) Look for good role models in magazines, especially 'slimming' type magazines, on television and in the newspapers. Think Slim: if they can do it – so can you.

- Co-operate with a slimming friend. This is fine if you support each other, and as long as you do not depend too much on each other.

  Avoid playing games such as: 'I'll have a cream cake if you will' and over-sympathising with each other.

- Get support. There is more about this in Part 2 (see page 247). You are entitled to support. Ask for it from spouse, friends, family, a professional counsellor, or from a self-help group.

- Do a 'sponsored slim' so that you help others while you motivate yourself.

- Create a 'slimming folder' where you save inspiring slimming stories/ pictures, inspiring words, or ideas. Read it through to re-motivate yourself.

- Find a garment that is presently too small, and hang it up somewhere in view. Whenever you pass it, think to yourself: 'I'm absolutely determined to get in that.'

  Try it on at intervals (not too often!) and notice happily how it fits a little better each time (don't be impatient). A 'Slimmer of the Year' from *Slimming* magazine bought herself a pair of lacy red bikini pants in a size 12 when she started slimming. At that stage they would only go over her ankles, but she slimmed into them. I bought a strapless evening dress two sizes too small, and slimmed into it.

  If you are heavy now, don't buy skirts or trousers in your 'large' size. It is a psychological signal that you don't expect to be slimmer, and it will almost certainly add to your chances of failure.

- Set targets. This is so important that it has been given a section all to itself, which follows next.

- Give rewards. Reward is a great motivator. Maybe you have a near one who will, if prompted, offer a treat to you if you lose your excess weight. But, it is just as good for you to offer rewards to yourself. The rewards don't have to be expensive, although you could put away all those coins which you used to squander on snacks and you'll be surprised how much 'reward money' you can accumulate.

Unfortunately, we have been conditioned to regard food as reward, as celebrations and food have been associated since our first birthday. Stop assuming that Reward equals food. If this is hard to change at first, reward yourself with 'quality' foods such as smoked salmon or prawns instead of chocolate. Think what you would regard as a reward: a massage, a sauna, a professional make-up lesson; a beauty shop session;

eyelashes dyed; new clothes; a trip out; a visit to a friend you don't often see.

**THINK SLIM**
Your thoughts can motivate – or de-motivate. It is your choice which thoughts you allow to dominate your mind.

## THINK SLIM MOTIVATION
### TO BE TAKEN IN DAILY DOSES

MOTIVATING MYSELF

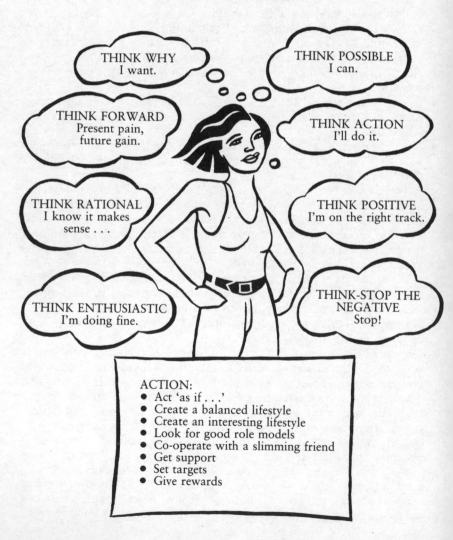

THINK WHY
I want.

THINK POSSIBLE
I can.

THINK FORWARD
Present pain,
future gain.

THINK ACTION
I'll do it.

THINK RATIONAL
I know it makes
sense . . .

THINK POSITIVE
I'm on the right track.

THINK ENTHUSIASTIC
I'm doing fine.

THINK-STOP THE
NEGATIVE
Stop!

ACTION:
- Act 'as if . . .'
- Create a balanced lifestyle
- Create an interesting lifestyle
- Look for good role models
- Co-operate with a slimming friend
- Get support
- Set targets
- Give rewards

# TARGET YOURSELF!
## If you don't know where you're going, you'll end up somewhere else

## WHY SET TARGETS?

A vital Think Slim Strategy for getting where you want to be (from fat to slim-fit) is target setting. Of course, target setting alone will not guarantee success, unless it is followed by plans and action. However, if you do not set targets, you make failure very likely. In fact, if you don't know where you're going, you'll end up somewhere else.

Target setting is used in the world of business for salespeople and for manufacturing, because it works. We can harness its power to our slimming.

Having a target gives you something specific to aim for, so that you are more likely to focus your attention on it. It prepares you mentally and emotionally to act in accordance with your aims. It is an expression that you are in charge of your life (self-empowered) and are taking decisions about what you will do.

## WHAT HELPS US TO REACH A TARGET?

Anyone (including you) can reach a Target:
  When you *know* what the Target is
  When the Target is *realistic*
  When you really *want* it
  When you *believe* that you can reach it
  When you *make sensible plans*
  When you *take action* to reach it
  When you *think positively (optimistically)* about it
  When you *accept* each set-back, and *bounce back*.

Let's consider each of the Target-setting 'whens':

1 **When you know what the target is.** Or, in the words of the old

song: 'if you don't have a dream, how you gonna have a dream come true?'

Know what you are aiming at. This need not necessarily be your ultimate weight-loss aim, for if you want to lose lots of weight it can seem so daunting that you go away and eat a cream cake to comfort yourself. So, at first, an intermediate target can be best. That first half stone, or stone, or 20 pounds (4, 6, 9 kilos) – it's your choice.

**2 When the Target is realistic.** 'I want to be slim for my holiday in four weeks!' announced Sallie, enthusiastically. But Sallie had over 2 stones/13 kilos to lose. She may 'want' to be slim for her holiday, and it would be very nice – but it is not realistic.

Unless she recognises that, she will become increasingly aware of her failure as her holiday draws near, and in the despair that she has created, she will slope off into corners with scones and jam for comfort and a 'Blow it!' attitude. She will then be the one trying to hide her even bigger roly-polies in an outsize pareo at the swimming pool. Sallie *can* be slimmer in four weeks, but needs to be realistic about what amount can be sensibly lost.

The realism of a weight-loss target also depends on how heavy you are now, and whether you are already slimming. The larger you are, the more likely you are to lose bigger amounts of weight regularly.

In the first week of your change to a slim-eating programme, you can expect to lose about 2 pounds/1 kilo. Some heavier people can lose more – maybe as much as 4–5 pounds/2–2½ kilos or up to 7 pounds/3 kilos. Of course, this is also dependent on how often you allow yourself to stray away from your Slim-fit Food and Drink Programme (see Step 6, page 167), so you need to be honest with yourself about your own likely dedication to following the eating and drinking guidelines.

It's OK to allow yourself some leeway for lapses and special occasions that might interrupt your weight losses.

**3 When you really want it.** Who are you slimming for? To please a spouse, to comply with a doctor – or for yourself, because you realise that you want the benefits of being slim-fit?

If you are slimming just for others, you are more likely to fail. If they disappoint or annoy you, you are likely to 'get back' at them by eating to spoil your slimming.

Check out your reasons for slimming. If it's not for yourself, think through the issues again. Why not, for you?

Occasionally, someone who says they are slimming for themselves and that they really want to be slim, have conscious (or unconscious) reasons to stay overweight that they are not admitting (or are not fully aware of). These are usually to do with their fears: fear of being slim (for it can seem a big and frightening change for some people); fear of more attention from others; fear of the increasing expectations from others; fear of sexuality (of being more attractive to the other sex, or of coping with a more-sexual relationship, fear of becoming promiscuous, or fears due to a traumatic history of sexual abuse or assault). Such fears can work against you to sabotage your efforts to slim, and are discussed in more detail in Step 2, Negative Wizards in yourself: 'Fear' (see page 103). If you have repeatedly tried to slim but seem to sabotage yourself each time, consider carefully the issues in that section.

**4 When you believe you can reach it.** This is a reiteration of Virgil: 'they can because they think they can' and has been fully explored under Step 3 on Motivation (see page 117). You need to believe; if you still doubt, re-read Step 3. Aim only for short-term targets at this stage, and don't think about your final desired slim weight.

**5 When you make sensible plans.** Plans, like Targets, must be realistic.
'I'll jog every day for half an hour!' If your plans are over-demanding and decided in a first flush of enthusiasm, they are guaranteed to fizzle out in the first week, the first rain-shower or the first attack of the blues. (Starting exercise should follow the build-up guidelines suggested, see page 210.)

Planning is needed to survive the slimming saboteurs; look back at the section on Negative Wizards and your completed Checklist (pages 111–113). (If you didn't complete it, plan when you will do so, and *do* it). Then plan how you are going to survive the saboteurs.

Planning is needed for you to begin your Slim-fit Food and Drink Programme:

See Step Six, Nourish Yourself (page 167). (Remember the story of the slimmer, who after two weeks of no weight loss, admitted to me that she 'hadn't read the programme yet'.) Then, plan your choices, and your shopping.

Alice was a planner, a tiny woman (in height, that is), with an elderly, smiley face and bright eyes, who set about planning as if it were a strategic battle. Each week's shopping, even each day's menus, were planned in advance, and written down. Alice enjoyed her planning, and never a week went by but Alice lost weight.

'I don't know how she does it!' marvelled another slimmer, half Alice's age. Alice did it by planning and then carrying out her plans. It's no use planning to eat a (low-fat) Lasagne but instead wolfing a steak and kidney pie followed by a piece of sponge cake. Alice reached her target weight, losing over 2 stones/13 kilos, and with her new approach stays slim and fit.

You don't have to be as meticulous as Alice (do it your way) but you do have to plan. Think Ahead, and Be Prepared.

There may be non-routine situations that occur in our lives that require some Slim Think-ahead planning, such as when you are decorating, driving long journeys, shopping, hospital visiting, or entertaining. None of these situations need sabotage your slimming unless you allow them to, or use them as a convenient excuse to over-indulge.

If you need food fast, it can be low calorie food: fruit, low-fat yoghurts, low-cal microwave meals, low-fat sandwiches in your freezer, tinned baked beans with microwave-baked potatoes; stir-fry veg; even a McDonald's hamburger costs only approx 250 calories. Earmark a local cafe/pub where you know they will serve you some low-fat foods, or choose the lowest calorie count options from an unfamiliar establishment, or ask for your sandwiches to be made up without butter.

You can train yourself into the good habit of planning how and what to eat, and it takes only a very very few minutes of your time when you are used to it.

If you are not doing this, why not? Don't play the 'yes, but' game, will you?

**6 When you take action to reach it.** Action must follow planning: remember Alice in the example above? The road to fat is paved with good intentions. And excuses. Think Slim: Make efforts not excuses.

You can keep your over-eating and your fat, but you can't keep your excuses for it. I know, and hopefully, by now so do you, that there is only one reason that we are overweight – that we over-eat for our unique body and our level of exercise.

It's our choice.

**7 When you think positively (optimistically) about it.** You have already read Step 1: Empower Yourself (page 17), haven't you? So you know all about this.

**8 When you accept each set-back, and bounce back.** Reaching a Target is never like getting from A to B in a nice neat straight line.

It can be more accurately represented like this:

Start............................................................................................ Target

The blips are the 'slip-ups' indicating where we fall by the wayside of the straight and narrow path, and deal with each set-back by bouncing back.

The diagram reminds me of a heart monitor print-out. It is interesting that the blips in such a print-out indicate that the patient is still alive. Your blips mean no more than that you are a living, normal sometimes-slipping-up human being. You will still reach your Target!

Make yourself a Think Slim card:

> If I have a Set-back
> I Bounce Back

## WHAT ARE YOUR TARGETS?

Think about your long-term target, and your first short-term target. Your long-term target can seem daunting, if you make it something like 'Lose 7 stones in weight/Lose 45 kilos in weight'. If you do wish to lose a large amount of weight, you could make your long-term target 'to become slim' and set no date, or set something like, 'by next summer' or 'Christmas'.

Jennie came to me for advice after she had fled from a diet group leader who had horrified her with the order that she had over 5 stones/32 kilos to lose. We set her targets at only half stone/3 kilo intervals. She is now 5 stones/32 kilos slimmer – on target – and has been for over three years.

Decide your weight aim for yourself. Please don't dash off to consult the dictatorial height and weight charts which are published in some slimming magazines and books. You *know* at approximately what weight you would feel comfortably slim – not 'perfect', nor 'thin'. You can always revise your target, later.

You may want to set other targets, besides weight-loss. One of mine was to wear a white bikini. And I did, but I was over 40 years old when I achieved it. If you're younger than that, don't postpone *your* pleasures. If you're older, it's never too late, and it's better late than never. For you, it doesn't have to be a bikini. Do it your way. Just remember, that this life Is Not A Dress Rehearsal.

Read, again, the 'What helps us to reach a Target' section before, and check that you understand and are following the advice.

## *PERSONAL WEIGHT-LOSS TARGET*

Setting yourself a fairly short-term weight-loss target is a good motivator, especially if you have a holiday, special occasion or celebration coming up in the not too distant future. To make it easier and keep your mind motivated, use a Personal Weight-loss Target plan as described below, together with completing a planner sheet as shown overleaf.

1 Check your diary and note six/eight/ten clear slimming weeks up to the special event or date that you have decided as the deadline for your Personal Weight-loss Target. Eight weeks is a good amount of time, but any of six, eight or ten weeks work well.

2 Note down in your diary the date you are going to start this Personal Target plan, and the date you are aiming for.
3 Think: decide on a realistic amount of weight you intend to lose during that period.
   - It is unlikely that you will lose an average of 2 pounds/1 kilo each week (unless you are very overweight, or just starting slimming) for each of eight weeks: for that period 14 pounds/6 kilos could be realistic.
   - *Don't* be over-ambitious.
   - Check if you have any celebrations/special events between now and then which you might allow to slow down your weight loss-progress.
   - Fill in the Personal Weight-loss Target sheet below. (The signature and date are to reinforce your commitment to achieving your target. Mark your weight loss on that sheet, every week.
   - Go for it!
   - Allow yourself a reward when you achieve the targeted weight.

## PERSONAL WEIGHT-LOSS TARGET
There are . . . . . . . . Think Slim weeks to . . . . . . . (event/date).

I *will* Think Slim every week.

My weight is now: _____

I *will* lose . . . . . . pounds/kilos by . . . . . . . . (date)

My weight will then be _____

Signed . . . . . . . . . . . . . . . . . . . . . . . . . . . . . . . . . . . .

Date: . . . . . . . . . . . . . . . . . . . . . . . . . . . . . . . . . .

WEEKLY RECORD OF WEIGHT LOSS

| Date | Weight | Weight Lost This Week | Weight Lost In Total | Comments |
|---|---|---|---|---|
| Week 1: | | | | |
| Week 2: | | | | |
| Week 3: | | | | |
| Week 4: | | | | |
| Week 5: | | | | |
| Week 6: | | | | |
| Week 7: | | | | |
| Week 8: | | | | |
| Week 9: | | | | |
| Week 10: | | | | |

You will find a further Weight-loss Record Sheet at the back of the book, on page 259. Or, you can use the Progress Chart on page 260.

Try using the target planner for long-term targets as well.

## REACHING YOUR TARGETS: THINK SLIM
- Read the Think Slim slogan below, and copy it on to a Think Slim card(s).
- Decide where you wish to display your card(s), and do so.
- Read it/them daily, as many times as possible. Danielle's young children daily read aloud her cards, to her, too. It helped their reading and their social education, for they need to learn how to be target setters in whatever they are aiming for in life, as well as helping her slimming.

```
I AM A PERSON WHO
   SETS A TARGET
    WORKS AT IT
        AND
      GETS IT
```

# ARM YOURSELF!
## When real life gets in the way

Despite our best preparations, Murphy's law reigns and real life has a nasty habit of interfering with our slimming. However, self-empowered slimmers realistically accept this as inevitable and do not dash off into a corner with a donut to rail against the world and comfort themselves. They look for solutions.

## SLIMMING AS A PROBLEM-SOLVING ACTIVITY

An obstacle to your slimming can be thought of as rather like a wall to be surmounted (or avoided), rather than as an excuse to indulge in the Negative Wizard Wooden Leg Syndrome: 'You can't expect me to slim, I've got . . .'

Norman Vincent Peale, an American who writes inspirational books on positive thinking, reminds us that the only people without problems are those in the cemetery. Problems are a sign of life! So, console yourself with that thought, and seek solutions.

If there is no solution, what you have is not a problem, but a Fact of Life. For example, I might see my small stature as a problem, because I could eat more if I were taller! My height isn't a problem. It's a Fact of Life. I can do nothing about it, so I need to accept it.

I accept it by using my Think Slim strategy. Catch that nega-thought: 'Just my luck! Nothing goes right for me! I'm fed up. I'll eat a . . .', and change it. 'Oh well, That's Life! Now, is there anything I can do about it?'

So, the self-empowered slimmer remembers the old proverb 'Where there's a will, there's a way', and looks for solutions, not excuses.

## OVERCOMING OBSTACLES

The pages that follow offer advice on overcoming common obstacles that beset slimmers. The 'obstacles' are arranged in alphabetical order, to assist you to locate them easily.

Every solution to every problem will not be found there, simply because each slimmer will have unique circumstances. However, you will find useful approaches, and you will be better equipped to find your own solutions, if you remember to cast away your Negative Wizard 'Yes, but' thoughts!

You could skim through these pages on first reading this book, so that you are familiar with the obstacles, and so you know where to look when any of them arise for you.

## OVERCOMING OBSTACLES: BOREDOM

'The Devil makes work for idle hands,' goes the old saying – and for slimmers the 'work' is always putting food into their mouths!

'It's boredom that's my problem,' diagnoses Carolyn. 'It's the evening, the children are in bed and I start to wander around, looking for something to eat.'

'Especially in the winter,' nods Cheryl, dismally, in agreement. 'In the summer I enjoy my gardening.'

Winter is the time to indulge in evening classes or at-home hobbies, rather than hot drinks and biscuits. This is going to sound tough, and it is, but it's true: you are the one who's bored, and it's you who's responsible for doing something about it.

'What do you do on Sunday afternoons?' I asked one of my slimmers.

'I stay in, and eat,' she admitted.

'What are your interests?' I enquired, of another.

She thought, for a long time. 'Well,' she declared, 'I worry a lot.' Such 'interests' are hardly the stuff of which exciting lives are made.

'My husband and I are both retired, and I realise that we've just been sitting at home, staring at each other, and eating,' confided Mary. A new way of life such as retirement, needs a new approach to life. No wonder many men die, fairly soon after retiring. They lose interest in living. The mind affects the body. People rust out before they wear out!

Try new hobbies or classes. Try one that you don't think you'll like – you may surprise yourself. Don't take up The Ostrich Position: 'I don't think I'll like it'. Once, I was press-ganged into taking an Astronomy class, and found, to my own surprise, a fascinating new interest.

Anna tried a photography class. Pete started singing in a choir. (Can't sing? Try lessons.) Bill started rock climbing. Carolann went to swimming lessons. You could try a Drama group. Make clocks. Public Speaking class. Gill writes to lots of penpals (the British magazine *Slimmer* offers penpals who are slimming; or you could advertise for someone who is slimming). Sarah kept her fingers out of food by teaching herself calligraphy. You could become a volunteer. Help handicapped children. Join a political party. Visit prisoners in jail. Offer to help the disadvantaged, maybe even overseas – you'll soon lose weight with a Third World diet! There is so much to do, if only we will kick-start ourselves.

We can learn from some young children, for they are hardly ever keen to eat because they are too busy doing, and playing and enjoying themselves living, to moon over food. Find the playful child in yourself, or your creative side.

Refuse to allow your life and your slimming to be blighted by boredom. Life is Not A Dress Rehearsal. This is the only life we can be sure that we have. Live now, for there is no 'later'!

Avoid the 'Yes, but' game, where every suggestion is met by you with, 'yes, but' and an excuse: 'I'd excrcise, but I've got a bad back', 'Swim? Yes, but I'm terrified of water!', 'Yes, but I've got two toddlers' . . . (See back to Negative Wizards, page 72.)

Two women who can be your role models are Janine and Val. Janine comes to my exercise class even though her back has a slipped disc, and after three months she is now amazingly more supple. But choose carefully your class and teacher; one who will be gentle with you whilst you be gentle with yourself. For back problems you could try the Alexander Technique. (See Useful Addresses Section, page 273.)

Val is wracked with arthritis, yet she attends my exercise class and finds it helpful. Losing weight also helps relieve the aches and pains from arthritis or back problems. Less weight, less aches and pains.

The Ultimate 'Yes, but' is 'Yes, but it's not that easy!', I know it isn't easy. Life isn't easy. I don't suggest that it is. I do say that most things can be done. Clearly, if you're over 40 and wannabe a professional ballet dancer, not only is it not easy, it's not possible. But with a bit of honesty, we can recognise what's impossible. The rest *is* possible.

Many women study for exams while caring for young children and/or doing a full time job (as I did). But you don't have to copy me, or anyone else. Design your own ladder to get out of the pit of boredom. Make your own rainbow in your life.

The answer to Boredom is always Action. Don't let Shirley Valentine's words be the epitaph on your tombstone: 'I've led such a little life. I've allowed myself to lead such a little life.'

Choose, change, and take action.


## COUNTERACT WITH THINK SLIM

- When you think: 'I'm bored, what shall I eat?', stop and change the thought to: 'I'm bored, what shall I DO?' Then, do!
- The responsibility for your boredom is yours. You are the one who is bored; you are the one to do something positive and practical about it (other than eat).
- If food is the 'only pleasure' in your life, look for other pleasures and change your life.
- Research 'What's On', or what volunteers are needed, at your local library.
- Ask others about the interests in their life – for ideas, not to play the 'Yes, but' game.
- Jot down ideas for new interests, and plans for what to do to get yourself started. Use the space overleaf:

Ideas                                    Action needed to Get Started

...................................................................................................

...................................................................................................

...................................................................................................

...................................................................................................

...................................................................................................

...................................................................................................

# OVERCOMING OBSTACLES: CHRISTMAS

### BEFORE CHRISTMAS: PREPARING YOURSELF FOR A STRESS-LESS YULE:

'Last year, I didn't enjoy Christmas because I was so overworked. On Christmas morning I still had to do my baking!' Susie sighed. Susie was suffering only from her own lack of organisation. Yet when I intimate that, she jumps to her own defence with some indignation. She is tempted to excuse herself with the 'Yes, but' game ('Yes, but there was so much to do – the children's concerts, the shopping, the official dinners').

Don't make excuses (nobody is castigating you); learn from your mistakes and Susie's.

Reduce your stresses (and the likelihood of comfort eating) by organising yourself, very early. Sonia had all of her presents and cards bought, sorted, wrapped and written by the beginning of December. Elaine is a teacher who always starts her Christmas shopping during the last week of her summer vacation. You don't have to follow these examples exactly, but they show you what's possible. For, Christmas arrives at the same date every year; yet every year, it seems to take many of us by surprise.

I didn't bake at all. The good supermarkets do it excellently on my behalf. It is not compulsory to bake. You are not less of a good wife or woman if you don't. Besides, baking means tasting for many slimmers, unless you resist by reminding yourself that every bit that goes into your mouth settles on your tum, hips and thighs.

### Pre-Christmas Preparation: tactics to help:

- Make lists. People to buy presents for; ideas of what to buy; card-list.
- Write out menu-plans for meals, along with the shopping needs.
- Plan when to shop, which weeks, days, times. Where to go, journeys arranged in the quickest order.
- When you shop for food, take your list and avoid wandering around fancy-packaged foodie temptations. If you go into a department store's food hall, always take a swift detour through the flimsy

underwear and posh frock departments; you need to remind yourself of the sleek goodies you'd like to wear to keep your mind off the excess food you'd like to gobble. (Having it all is an impossible dream.)

- Preparing Others: prepare your family and friends, well in advance, by writing a Note to Santa to let them know what you would like – and *not* like – for Christmas presents. Even young children can be encouraged to be considerate to your wants and avoid foodie presents for you.

**Your final, essential Think Slim preparation by Christmas Eve:** make a note on card (large and left somewhere prominently!) for yourself:

**On 27th December, turn to the Think Slim book, page 141.**

**Slimming yourself before Christmas.** Many people are highly motivated to lose weight before Christmas so they can look better for the celebration season. So, while determination is high, it's a good time to make a special effort.

Committing yourself to a Christmas weight loss target is an excellent way of maximising your good slimming results. Ninety per cent of the slimmers in my group attain their promised target of weight losses this way before Christmas. You can choose whether to make your special slim-plan start six/eight/ten weeks before Christmas. Refer back to the Weight-loss Target plan on page 131–3.

**Christmas weight loss target**

1 Check your diary and note six/eight/ten clear slimming weeks up to Christmas.

2 Note down in your diary the date you are going to start this Christmas plan.

3 Think: decide on a realistic amount of weight you intend to lose during that period.

- Don't be over-ambitious: 2 pounds/1 kilo per week is the maximum average you could expect.
- Check if you have many pre-Christmas Christmas Celebrations.
- Fill in a Christmas weight loss target sheet, as on page 132.
- Mark your weight loss on that sheet, every week.
- Go for it!
- Allow yourself a reward when you achieve it.

**Pre-Christmas Christmas celebrations.** For many of us, Christmas celebrations begin early, even as far back as November, when 'Christmas' functions from work, friends, charity fund-raising, and other organisations begin to be held. These accumulating celebrations can soon accumulate fat on your hips and what's-its, so that you will look like a pudding come Christmas unless you employ Think Slim strategies to survive.

## COUNT THE CALORIE COST OF CHRISTMAS EATING
Prepare yourself with knowledge of what Christmas fare can cost in calories. Try this Quiz, then check the answers on page 265.

How many calories (approx) in these festive foods?

|  | Approx calories |
|---|---|
| 1 oz/28 g stuffed olives | ..................... |
| 1 mince pie | ..................... |
| 1 peanut | ..................... |
| 1 oz/28 g peanuts, roasted and salted | ..................... |
| 1 oz/28 g roast turkey (no skin) | ..................... |
| 1 oz/28 g roast duck (no skin) | ..................... |
| 1 large roast potato | ..................... |
| 5 oz/150 g Christmas pudding | ..................... |
| 1 oz/28 g brandy butter | ..................... |
| 3½ oz/100 g Christmas cake | ..................... |
| 1 luxury chocolate | ..................... |
| 1 oz/28 g shortbread | ..................... |
| 1 oz/28 g grapes (black or green) | ..................... |
| 1 tangerine (c. 3½ oz/100 g) | ..................... |
| 1 oz/28 g fresh dates | ..................... |
| 1 oz/28 g dates, dried with stones | ..................... |
| 1 oz/28 g brazil nuts (shelled) | ..................... |
| 1 oz/28 g walnuts (shelled) | ..................... |
| 1 oz/28 g chestnuts (shelled) | |

Answers on page 265.

## COUNTERACT PRE-CHRISTMAS CELEBRATIONS WITH THINK SLIM
- Many early events will have traditional Christmas menus. So, check out the 'Count the Calorie Cost of Christmas' quiz so that you are aware of what you might be eating.
- Think Slim: Think Before You Eat a Thing!
- Before you eat, *always* ask yourself and answer the fundamental Think Slim question: 'Is It Worth Its Calories?'
- For various possible approaches to your Pre-Christmas eating out, refer to the 'Eating Out' pages of this section (see page 143).

## AT CHRISTMAS
The self-empowered slimmer can choose how to deal with eating over Christmas from these alternative approaches.

1 **The 'Christmas won't crack me' calorie counter.** If you are very determined, you could count your calories over the three main Christmas

days, allowing yourself a pre-decided number of little-bits-of-what-you-fancy extras to eat; say, no more than 500 calories for a woman or 800 for a man over the Basic 1000 Calories a day. Then resume a basic day afterwards. You should manage to hold your weight stable or minimise weight gain.

**2 The 'To hell with it – I'm enjoying Christmas!' uninhibited approach.** If, when you read those words, your thoughts are already screaming 'yes, yes please!' then you are still in the grip of Excess-ism, and you need to turn to the 'Negative Wizards in yourself – Excess-ism' section (see page 64) to learn about defeating your own sabotaging attitude.

For this approach will do maximum damage to your slimming, and probably upset your stomach. However, it's your choice, and maybe you've not been Thinking Slim long enough to be wiser yet.

Charlotte was one who took this 'over-eat now, fat later' approach. She added over 10 pounds/4½ kilos in weight, and, having only just reached the target weight loss she had set herself, she found it took her until Easter to remove it again. Fatter, sadder and wiser, she said: 'never again!' The next year she tried approach Number 3.

**3 The 'Moderation will do nicely, thank you' style.** Think Slim applies: 'We don't have to eat and drink too much to have a good time.'

Moderation means eating those items that you really want and that you have answered yes to the question: 'is it worth its calories?' (You have checked through the 'Calorie cost of Christmas' quiz to make you aware, haven't you?)

Moderation has had a bad press. It's been marketed as boring, and only excess is depicted as fun. Clearly, this is irrational thinking that has brainwashed our society. We need to refute it – moderation is the magnificent way. It means having the nearest you can get to the best of both worlds, that is, getting and staying slim plus still enjoying your food. Do a bit of enjoyable algebra: learn, and draw on a Think Slim card the Moderation Equation:

$$\text{MODERATION} = \text{GETTING/STAYING SLIM} + \text{ENJOYING YOUR FOOD}$$

With this approach during Christmas, you will probably add up to 5 pounds/2 kilos or so to your weight. Some of that will be water-gain not fat, and so will soon disappear from the scales if you immediately start the after Christmas Think Slim strategies, shown below.

## AFTER-CHRISTMAS THINK SLIM STRATEGIES
### DEC 27TH!
Christmastide has come and gone. You have probably gained weight, but

that's OK. You've no need to feel guilty, because you chose to indulge yourself, and are prepared to pay the price (aren't you?).

The worst danger is allowing your Christmas eating to drag on; if you greedily over-indulge in twelve days of festive foodie revels, you will have tremendous difficulties in removing your fatty results. You need to get 'back to normal' with your Think Slim strategies as well as your eating and drinking (maybe with a thankful sigh from your digestive system), right now.

- Check your weight. If you have not gained weight, congratulate yourself! If you have gained weight, don't start berating yourself, or thinking despairing thoughts.

First, write down your weight-gain, here: _____

Next, set yourself a new (realistic) target to get rid of the festive flab:
  'I shall lose .... lbs/kg by ...... (date).
  Think Slim: 'I've had a good Christmas-time. Now I'll get off that festive flab!'

- Cut back *wisely* on your eating. (Check the Food and Drink section, page 184, for details.)
- Ban alcohol for at least five days.
- Do some sensible extra exercise, such as 20 minutes each day of walking, swimming or cycling at a pace to suit your current level of fitness.
- Remove 'left-over' foodie temptations
    – into the freezer
    – into the bin
    – into the local orphanage, or hospital, or . . .
    – anywhere except into your mouth!
- Start to think about New Year Resolutions (see the appropriate section of this book, page 127, to help you).

## OVERCOMING OBSTACLES: EATING OUT

Eating out can be a great challenge to your slimming. In surveys, men often cite eating out as a major cause of their excess weight and difficulty in losing it. However, whether you are eating out for business or leisure, there are different approaches to avoid over-eating. The self-empowered slimmer chooses the way that best suits her/him.

**1 Forget the Slimming! Have It All!** This may work for certain slimmers. Ask yourself the following questions. If you answer yes to every one, then you should be able to use this approach successfully.

  Are you: (a) someone who eats out *rarely* (say, less than once in six weeks)?
  (b) prepared to accept any resulting weight gain without getting discouraged?

(c) sure that you will start back on your wise ways of slimming immediately?

If so, the very occasional over-indulgence should not ruin your slimming. However, think carefully and honestly whether this way is for you.

**2 Stay With It! Keep to Your Food and Drink Programme Guidelines.** Do this by choosing only those foods in the (approximate) right quantities that you would if you were eating at home, or by calculating the calorie total (calculators allowed!).

Obviously, this is effective – if you are willing to exercise the self-control to do it. If so, congratulations, and carry on!

**3 'Indulge and Make Up'.** It is only those who over-indulge who bulge. Think Slim: we don't have to eat and drink too much to have a good time. Moderation is the magnificent style.

You can indulge on a moderate, planned scale, and 'make up' by reducing your calorie intake, on both the day before and the day after the meal. This allows you to indulge rather than over-indulge, and only eat truly scrumptious food that's worth its calories! (Think Slim: Is It Worth Its Calories?) This is effective if it is planned, and kept to.

Remember that restaurants often increase calorie content by their preparation of food, such as frying meat, adding cream to sauces, using high-fat salad dressings.

Then, afterwards, no backsliding on the 'balancing' of calories!

This method is my favourite. Sometimes it can be amusing.

'Oh, you've forgotten your roast potatoes, Eve,' Peter commented at a buffet. He added, solicitously, 'I'll go and get some for you.'

'No, thanks,' I replied cheerfully, as he rose and picked up my plate. 'I don't want any.' I held on to my plate.

He pulled. 'Of course you do. You must have some delicious roast potatoes.'

I tugged my plate back. 'No, thanks!'

The plate hovered precariously over the table as we tugged it between us, as in a pantomime farce with its 'Yes you do', 'No I don't' script.

'Peter, I'm having a great time and my happiness doesn't depend on having roast potatoes. I'd rather have your company', I finished, and Peter, mystified, capitulated.

For me, roast potatoes are simply not worth their 200 calories-a-chunk price. But I'll not be missing the lemon meringue pie afterwards (if it's good enough!).

**4 Eat a little of everything.** It has been rumoured that the Queen, and Princess Diana, use this system. Judging by their figures, it works – but only if 'a little' really *is* a little'!

**5 Choose the lowest-calorie dishes available.** A useful system, and you need to learn which choices are 'cheapest' in their calorie cost.

This way of dealing with eating out is Katherine's favourite. Her figure is now as sleek as her brunette bobbed hair (nearly two stones less of flab than there always used to be). At a formal dinner, her next-door neighbour, an attractive man, must have been watching her choice of menu. He commented drily at the end of the meal: 'Now I know why you look like you do, and why my wife looks like she does.' (There's no need for Katherine to describe the 'look' of the wife, is there?)

Learn which are the lower-calorie dishes (see page 174–5 for suggestions).

Be an assertive customer. You are entitled to ask the chef to provide plainly cooked versions of meat, fish or vegetables, with no added butter on serving.

## EATING OUT – CALORIE CHOICES
If you wish to choose the foods with the lowest calorie costs, this chart will guide you:

| CHOOSE | AVOID |
| --- | --- |
| **STARTERS** | |
| Melon | Avocado |
| Prawns | Mushrooms in batter |
| Smoked salmon | Pâté |
| Tuna | Creamy soups |
| Crudites, but not the 'dip' | |
| **MAIN COURSE** | |
| Poultry | Duckling |
| White fish | Red meat |
| Fresh salmon | Cream sauces |
| Lobster | Pastry dishes |
| Lean pork | Quiche |
| | Suet puddings |
| | Mayonnaise dressing |
| | Oily salad dressing |
| **DESSERTS** | |
| Sorbets | Rich ice cream |
| Meringue | Gateaux/cakes |
| Fresh fruit | Pies/pastries |
| Unsweetened fresh fruit salad | Fritters |
| Low fat cheese | Full fat cheeses |
| None! | Steamed puddings |
| | Cream |
| | Creamy chocolates |

For more calorie information (in Britain), you could consult Slimming Magazine's publication *Your Greatest Calorie Guide to Eating Out.* Ask your newsagent or bookseller.

## COUNTERACT WITH THINK SLIM
- Choose the method that works best for you.
- Avoid salad bars, unless you refuse the high-calorie mayonnaise-dressed salads, or take your own low-calorie salad dressing with you in a small container.
- Do make the effort to get *any* establishment to accommodate you! *You* are the customer, and many managers are delighted to assist, if only you will ask! The problem of over-eating is often with slimmers themselves, who are only too pleased to find an excuse to over-indulge! You won't, will you?
- If you are 'Business eating' often, you may be able to frequent a particular restaurant, which will then become familiar with you and more responsive to your needs.
- Avoid or limit alcohol.
- 'I've paid for it so I've got to eat it' is Think Fat! Think Slim: If you've paid for it you can do anything you like with it! (Eat it, leave it, take it home, throw it at your companion . . .)
- Think Slim: Regard the occasion, and your companions, as your main pleasures, rather than the food and drink! Remember the Think Slim phrase: 'We don't have to eat and drink too much to have a good time'.

## OVERCOMING OBSTACLES: FAILING DAYS
'I've had a dreadful day . . . eat eat eat . . . one thing after another . . .!' Gil moaned to herself as she climbed wearily and heavily into bed.

Occasionally, despite your best intentions and preparations, you are likely to have slimming Failing Days. It is important that you know how to deal with the close of such a day, so that one Failing Day does not become a week or a month or a lifetime.

## COUNTERACT WITH THINK SLIM
At the end of such a day:
- Refuse to insult yourself as hopeless or a failure.
- Remind yourself that you are only human, and that you are entitled to be imperfect occasionally.
- Think Slim: 'No one is a failure until they give up trying.'
- Briefly, review where you went wrong during the day:
  (a) What were the outside triggers for over-eating? (An invitation, an insult, a person, the smell of food, the sight of it, etc.)
  (b) What were your trigger thoughts that encouraged or allowed you to over-eat?
  (c) Next time, what shall I think – and do – instead?

- Remind yourself that you can fight better another time because you will prepare yourself better. This review will help you to be better prepared the next time those triggers tempt you.
- Say goodnight to your Failing Day by dismissing it with: 'Never mind! Tomorrow is another day and I'm absolutely determined to make it a better day.'
- Before you go to sleep, recite some of your positive Think Slim thoughts to yourself, such as:
  Life's Too Short to Live It Fat.
  Others slim successfully. If They Can Do It So Can I.
  I'm absolutely determined to slim . . . I'm absolutely determined to slim . . . I'm . . .
  Successful Slimmers Make It Happen. I'm a Successful Slimmer. (Yes, you are. You've lost weight already, haven't you?)
- Tell yourself that as soon as you awake in the morning you will repeat some of your Think Slim positive thoughts.
- Take some slow, deep breaths (in through your nose and out through your mouth), and repeat your favourite Think Slim positive thoughts to yourself as you begin to drift off to sleep . . .

## OVERCOMING OBSTACLES: HOLIDAYS

Welcome and wonderful as our holidays are, they can be obstacles to slimming. Holidays, as with eating out, can be dealt with in different ways, and the slimmer needs to decide which is the best way for her/him. Also, different types of holiday come with their own built-in advantages and disadvantages for the slimmer.

If your holiday is a once-a-year week or fortnight fling, you may think that you want to take a holiday from slimming too, and throw your calorie caution to the winds. However, this attitude indicates that you are still trapped by that old diet-think; that you are not yet regarding your new eating habits as a lifestyle for a lifetime.

Certainly, it is possible to choose to over-indulge on a moderate scale on your holiday, but still apply some of your fundamental Think Slim thoughts, particularly: 'Is It Worth Its Calories?'

Zena recently returned from a two-week holiday in Spain with no extra weight at all. She explained: 'I just kept asking myself "Is it worth its calories?" and to be honest, the starters and desserts weren't very interesting, so I didn't have them.'

So, Think Slim: 'If the food's not fabulous, don't waste the calories.'

Some people are able to take lots of holidays. For example, Vera and her husband go away in their caravan frequently throughout the summer. They usually cater for themselves and so can keep to their Think Slim cooking principles, and their slimming can continue nomadically. If, however, you are travelling abroad where you suspect that your favourite low-cal substitutes may not be available, then you need to prepare a list of items to take with you, such as low-fat spread, crispbreads, high fibre cereal, low fat cheese.

If you take frequent holidays or business trips, you need to think carefully in advance about how you will deal with the eating. Read the 'Eating Out' section to find ideas for surviving, and decide on your own strategy.

My husband and I always choose hotels that have leisure and fitness facilities, and every day we swim, use the exercise bike and electric jogger, and my husband uses the weight machines. It is possible to find such hotels in almost all parts of the globe, if you make it a priority to look for them. They are helpful in that you can indulge yourself a little more with eating without paying such a heavy price in weight gain. You should not, of course, throw yourself into an unfamiliar, demanding exercise programme while on holiday, or you might prompt a heart attack instead of weight loss.

George is a stay-slim travelling businessman who also routinely stays at hotels where such fitness facilities are provided. He finds the effects of business stresses are also lessened when he works out before breakfast and again in the evening, and he can enjoy a relaxing sauna, too. (A sauna is of no use in promoting weight loss; any immediate weight loss due to sweating is almost immediately regained; fat cannot be 'burned off' by the heat of a sauna.)

Even if your hotel has no fitness facilities, extra exercise in the form of swimming and walking can often be enjoyed nearby.

'When I come back from my hols, I get the post-holiday blues,' grumbled Cherie. 'Ordinary life seems so dull, and it seems such a long time to the next holiday . . and I've got used to eating more goodies and I cheer myself up with a bit of this and that . . .'

I can identify with her feelings, but I don't have them any more.

Where do those post-holiday blues come from? Our post-holiday thoughts, that's where. So, determine to change your thoughts, and your actions. I always save some 'holiday money' to spend after I've returned from holiday, so that I have an outing planned during the come-home week to look forward to. This works wonders.

Also, think about your 'ordinary' life; perhaps it is too dull. A cream donut is always enticing, but it becomes almost irresistible if life is dreary. You can change your life, in both little and big ways. Perhaps now is a good time to think about what you would like to change, and then how you can make a start on changing it. Refuse to play the Cinders Game, waiting for a fairy godmother to do it all for you.

On the last day: As you start to pack up your belongings, pack up your over-indulgent holiday thinking and eating habits.

Return to your home Think Slim routines. Start to imagine yourself, back in your usual routine. Plan what you are going to do when you get home; and plan what you will be eating the next day. (Lots of fresh fruit to relieve your over-indulged digestion?) You could vow to ban alcohol for at least five days to also relieve your body.

Think of something interesting to do during your homecoming week: a new class to try; a friend to ring or see; somewhere to explore; a new hairstyle; a visit to a beauty shop; a new exercise class or routine to start; some voluntary work. Think positive, act positive.

Remind yourself to turn back to this book for inspiration.

**On your return**: Now that your indulgent holiday is over, you need to get 'back to normal' with your eating and drinking. Don't be tempted to think 'I'll start tomorrow', for you know that you need to start right now, or an indulgent holiday bulge or two will become permanent bulk.

Don't let yourself fall into 'poor me' thinking as you start back into your normal lifestyle. Think about how you've enjoyed your indulgent holiday, and now you are prepared to cheerfully pay the price: weight gain and the effort to remove it.

'Back to normal' means back to your Think Slim habits as well as eating and drinking habits as advised in the Food and Drink Programme.

So: weigh yourself. If you haven't gained any weight (or if you've lost a bit), congratulate yourself! Then think about setting your next sensible weight loss target.

Otherwise:
- Write down the weight you've gained, here . . . . . .
- Set a new, realistic, Target
   I will lose . . . . . . by . . . . . . . . . (date)
- Repeat to yourself, often:
   I am a person who
   Sets a target,
   Works at it
   and Gets it.
- Plan your eating; be stringent for a week; weigh your portions; indulge in no extra 'little of what you fancy' for a week.

Zoe gained 4 pounds/2 kilos during her holiday; she lost it within two weeks.

'This is the first time I've ever managed that,' she said, pleased. 'Before, I've always just carried on my holiday eating. Now I've really got into the way of thinking.'

Zoe has mastered a useful technique – a thinking one to help her for all the holidays in her lifetime.

You can too.

## OVERCOMING OBSTACLES: MENOPAUSE

'It seemed to creep up on me, without me knowing what it was,' began Edith. 'I'd been feeling generally more tired than before, and vaguely depressed for no apparent reason; losing weight seemed more difficult than it had ever been. My skin was drier and flakier, and my sex life had been affected by that 'drying up' process; even when I felt aroused, it was as if my body was separate, and it didn't respond as usual.

'Then, at 46 years old, I started with the flushes,' she continued. 'I had heard of flushes, of course, but I had no idea what they would feel like – and it was an awful shock! My clothes were soaked wet with them, and I had never expected so many each day! It was embarrassing to be at work. Once I had to go to the Ladies room and have a total strip wash before an important meeting. My periods hadn't changed at all. But, I was waking up about five o'clock each morning, in a sweat, with my heart pounding as if it would burst. It felt quite frightening. I was even more tired from this lack of sleep . . . Life was becoming a real drag.'

If Edith's distressing experiences are familiar to you, you don't have to suffer in silence. Edith decided to visit her doctor.

'He insisted that I needed anti-depressant tablets,' she said, 'and I allowed him to prescribe them. Yet I didn't think they were right – I wasn't suffering from depression.'

Edith felt no better, and started to do her own research in the library on HRT, the Hormone Replacement Therapy that alleviates the menopausal changes. She received information from The Amarant Trust, a charitable body set up to spread the word on HRT. (See page 273 for contact information.)

'What I read convinced me that I wanted to try it,' she explained, 'so I went back to my doctor, taking my folder on HRT information and I told him that I felt no better, didn't want to continue on the anti-depressant tablets, and that I wanted to try HRT.'

Faced with Edith's positive approach, the doctor agreed, and the dreaded flushes subsided within two days and disappeared within five.

'It was like magic. It was absolutely marvellous!' she enthused. 'Not just the flushes gone, but depression lifted, my energy returned, the vaginal moistness starting to flow again . . .'

Edith needed some trial-and-error adjustments to her prescription, and altogether she tried four types of medication before finally settling to one that totally suited her.

She explains: 'The first tablet wasn't quite strong enough. Some flushes returned, but I put on no weight. The second dosage held off the flushes, but I did gain half a stone/3 kilos in weight. Also, I began to have a migraine each month. So I tried another brand, and the migraines disappeared, but the weight was persisting. Then I tried a smaller dosage of the same brand and, Eureka, it's just right! My slimming worked fine, and I'm staying easily at my target weight.'

It's almost like the story of The Three Bears: too much, too little, and finally Just Right. An important moral of Edith's story is that she persisted to find the brand and dosage that really suited her. Another slimmer, Alice, tried HRT for about one month and decided it didn't suit her, and gave up. This is not the way for a self-empowered woman to react. If at first you don't succeed . . .

Some women have a hormone-releasing patch (stuck onto the skin and replaced every few days) instead of tablets, others have an implant under the skin. Trials are sometimes needed; be persistent.

**'The Change' – what changes?** As women grow older, their ovaries produce less and less of the female hormones, oestrogen and progesterone, which finally results in the total loss of fertility and 'the menopause'. (The word 'menopause' literally means 'cessation of the periods', but the word is often used colloquially to mean all the changes connected to that reduction of the female hormones. The proper name for the time leading up to the cessation of the periods is 'climacteric' but it is not used very often.)

Changes occur as the body adjusts to the up-and-down levels of the hormones: hot flushes, early awakening with heart palpitations, dryness of skin, thinning of the hair, drying up of secretions in the vagina, thinning of the vaginal walls, associated depression, lack of ability to concentrate, and mood swings. Quite understandably, anxiety and loss of confidence often also result from experiencing these physical changes.

The severity of these changes varies between women; some women are fortunate and experience very little problem, while others find it an extremely difficult period in their lives.

**What exactly is HRT?** It is Hormone Replacement Therapy, the replacement of the woman's natural female hormones, oestrogen and progesterone, by prescribed 'artificial' hormones. Their effect is to hold off the menopause and its changes. Usually the woman still has a period each month (although a new product which avoids this has recently arrived).

**The Benefits of HRT.** HRT can restore a woman to the state she has been enjoying while her body has been producing female hormones. HRT stops the problems associated with 'The Change': hot flushes, dryness of skin; drying up of the vagina. It also reduces bone loss. After the menopause, when no more female hormones are being produced, about 25 per cent of women suffer from osteoporosis, or 'brittle bones' which is thought to cause the hump-backed 'little old lady' syndrome, and also fractures of the hip or limbs. Heart attacks and breast cancers are much more common in women who are no longer producing oestrogen than in younger women, and it is thought that HRT can help to prevent both.

**Any Side Effects?** Some dosages may increase weight, but not substantially. However, changing brands and/or dosage can alleviate this.

There may be some 'pre-menstrual' symptoms, such as swollen breasts, or water retention. (Deal with these as suggested in the Pre-menstrual advice section.)

**Any Dangers?** No prescribed medicine can be guaranteed absolutely safe; we accept some risk in taking anything. Doctors may prefer not to prescribe HRT if there is a family history of ovarian or breast cancer; but your doctor should discuss this with you.

**Alternative Views.** There are always alternative views. I read once of a gynaecologist who said that women should not be told how good HRT was, or they would all want it, and how expensive that would be!

One woman doctor is quoted as believing that menopausal discomfort is merely a preoccupation of middle-class woman, brought on by suggestion from reading too much about it. My message to her is don't dismiss it till you've suffered it! Her generalised view is both patronising and insulting. If you are suffering, and this is the view in your doctor's surgery, change doctors.

Some commentators argue that Japanese and Indian women don't seem to suffer, so it must all be in our imagination. It is poor science to assume that what is usual for one race is also usual for another race living a different lifestyle. Tell them you are pleased for the Japanese and Indians, but it is irrelevant to your situation, here and now.

Some women play the martyr game and think they Should suffer; others think that they Should be brave; a few think that women's troubles Should be endured. A self-empowered Think Slimmer will *dismiss* such irrational 'should-bes' and remember that This Is Not A Dress Rehearsal. Live now – there is no 'later'. Play no 'martyr' nor 'should-be' games.

## OVERCOMING MENOPAUSAL PROBLEM CHANGES

- If you are suffering, don't delay. Find out more information about HRT for yourself (see Useful Addresses) and then make an appointment with your doctor.
- Before you go to see your doctor, prepare yourself. Take your 'research' information with you; write down any questions you want answering; decide what symptoms you must report, and write them down so you won't miss any out. Be open about any sexual difficulties you experience. (You could say: 'Nowadays, my body doesn't give enough sexual lubrication', or 'Sexual intercourse is painful' – just describe what is true for you.) If you feel embarrassment, reduce it by practising the sentences before you go.

    If you are a bit nervous of insisting on what you want, practise your 'lines' again before you set off. For example: 'I've thought about it, and I want to try HRT.'
- If your doctor refuses to prescribe HRT, consider changing your doctor, or going to a women's clinic for a consultation. Be assertive. Whose menopausal problems are they, anyway?
- Don't say (or think): 'It's because I'm taking HRT,' as an excuse for your over-eating habits when you are overweight, or for not losing weight when in fact you are not being careful enough. If your HRT

dosage is causing weight gain, arrange with your doctor to change the brand/dosage.

**A Note:**
It is not too late to start taking HRT if you are over menopausal problems but are worried about Osteoporosis, especially if there is a family history of it.

## OVERCOMING OBSTACLES: PARTIES!

Parties can be a great challenge to the slimmer. The groaning buffet table can leave you groaning next time on the scales, because it is often even more expensive in calories than it appears. However, forewarned is forearmed, and these Think Slim Strategies will help your slimming.

### SURVIVE YOUR PARTIES
- Don't 'starve' yourself all day before a party; you will be so hungry you may 'binge'.
- Have a day of light eating both the day before, the day of, *and* the day after your party. Have more fruit and vegetables than usual and less of the carbohydrates such as bread, potato, pasta and rice.
- Do Think ahead. Decide beforehand whether you will indulge in alcohol, and if so, how much. (Too much alcohol uses too many calories, dissolves your Think Slim reasoning-power, and prompts too much eating.)
- Make alcohol 'shorts' into long drinks by adding low-cal mixers. Add calorie-free soda water to wine to make a 'spritzer'. Or, alternate a 'short' with a non-alcoholic drink.
- Dance away the night and the calories. It's enjoyable and minimises time for food and drink.
- There is no need to cut out your favourite foods, but do eat *less* of them.
- Refuse to eat something of everything just because it's on offer.
- Think of your main enjoyment as the company and the socialising, rather than the food and drink.

### GIVING A PARTY?
Remember these Think Slim Strategies too:
- Use low-calorie alternatives wherever possible when catering.
- Have low-cal 'dips' with raw vegetable crudites available, instead of nuts, crisps, etc.
- Avoid pork pies, sausage rolls, sausages-on-sticks. They're predictable and boring as well as fattening.
- Offer visually appealing party food, such as colourful rice salads; various coleslaws with low-cal dressings; tiny rolled-up sandwiches; chicken drumsticks; rolled lean meats rather than filled bread rolls. Think about presentation; decorate the food and the table.

- Put aside a plate of carefully chosen lower-calorie food for yourself beforehand – then eat no more.
- Have low-cal mixers available, at least for yourself.
- Provide some attractive low-cal, non-alcoholic cocktails.
- Put food and drink in a separate room from the dancing/socialising – it's less tempting.

### GOING TO A PARTY?
More Think Slim Strategies:
- Take low-cal mixers with you.
- Choose mostly the lower-calorie food, and *stop* any intruding little thoughts of 'poor deprived me'.
- Avoid second helpings from the buffet, even if others do. Think how greedy they are.

### FINALLY:
- Take time beforehand to make the most of your slimmer appearance, and let yourself enjoy it.
- Repeat the Think Slim slogan: 'We don't have to eat and drink too much to have a good time!'

## OVERCOMING OBSTACLES: THE PATTER OF TINY FEET

### 1 AFTER PREGNANCY:
'It was pregnancy that did for me!' explained Kerry. 'I was slim till I had my two children, but I put on weight each time and it never really went . . .'

It is never actually pregnancy that 'did it'; but 'eating for two' is a super self-indulgent excuse for having a nine-month fling with food that results in a swollen shape that stays around long after baby has left the womb. Next, the change of life from woman to woman/mother is a shock that sends most of us reeling in the direction of the biscuit barrel while we learn to adjust.

The first step on the road back to slim-fitness is to stop blaming pregnancy. If we continue to think of pregnancy as 'The Cause', as if it had some special power to balloon our weight permanently, we shall feel powerless to reverse the process. Then we shall *be* powerless to act. Remember the 'Think – Feel – React' Diagram?

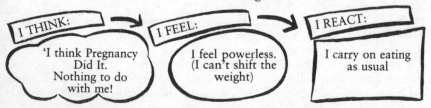

I THINK: 'I think Pregnancy Did It. Nothing to do with me!'

I FEEL: I feel powerless. (I can't shift the weight)

I REACT: I carry on eating as usual

## COUNTERACT WITH THINK SLIM
- Use the Thought-stopping Technique whenever you think your overweight can be blamed on pregnancy. Say STOP THIS! to yourself.
- Re-think, and accept that over-eating during pregnancy meant overweight afterwards. Think Slim: We are overweight because we over-eat.
- Read the following sections about coping with children, to help you.

## 2  AT HOME ALL DAY WITH . . .
'I'm at home all day with Laura. I nibble biscuits when she nibbles, and I have to finish up her left-overs. Then she's so demanding that I get exhausted and fed up, so I eat to cheer myself up, and to give me more energy!' Judi's tale of slimming woe is a common one for women whose real life problem is lovable but stressful toddlers at home.

Being at home all day with toddlers is a demanding situation, but it doesn't inevitably mean slimming failure. What it needs is some Slim Thinking about how you are managing yourself, your toddlers and your life.

Unfortunately, no one ever teaches us how best to tackle motherhood. Just because Mother Nature dished out the necessary equipment it is assumed that the skills are also natural. Equipment comes naturally, skills don't. Ante-natal classes teach us relaxation techniques for coping with labour, but no one teaches survival skills for mothers. Our culture pressures us to be Mrs Perfect Mum but does not admit the impossibility of that job description.

First, let's consider the specific situations faced by an at-home mum (or Dad) like Judi: 'I nibble biscuits when she nibbles . . .'

Contrary to popular myth and the pressure of the consumer industry, it is *not* compulsory for children to nibble biscuits. You will not be disqualified from the 'Mum of the Year Award' if you do not provide biscuits. Nor crisps; nor chips; nor treacle puds. Of course, what may be happening is that a Negative Wizard is lurking inside you and tempting you to excuse your fat-eating by blaming your good mothering. So, if you find yourself strongly believing that children must have fatty munchie treats, turn to the section in this book on 'Negative Wizards in Yourself' (see page 66) and spend some time examining your own attitude honestly. You can keep your fat-eating and your fat, but you can't kid me that you have a good mothering excuse as well.

Ilona is a slim-fit mum who successfully banned biscuits and other high-calorie kiddie treats for her two boys. The boys are now 14 and 16 years old, and they have managed to grow up into 'normal', bright, boisterous, aggravating, loveable, charming, slim and healthy teenagers despite it.

Toddlers don't need a hand permanently dipping down into packets and up into mouths. If they are physically hungry for a snack, let them eat fruit. They don't like it? Your baby is not born with a natural lust for technicolor sweeties, chunky chocolate or barbecue-flavoured crisps (nor were you!), but baby acquires a taste according to how you teach her or him. Children will eat fruit if it's the only alternative to being hungry. If they refuse, that's fine: they won't starve between now and their next meal. They might even, with the spur of real hunger, enjoy it more.

If you train children into a state of permanent snacking and an addiction to high calorie goodies, you are condemning them to life in the fat lane or the diet trap, or into buying this book twenty years from now and having to re-educate themselves painfully, just as you and I have had to do. Is that good mothering?

**Left-Overs**: Let's check what else Judi said. 'I have to finish up her left-overs . . .' *Have to*? Really? Who insists it's compulsory? (Or is this another Negative Wizard in yourself – just a good excuse to indulge in little extras?)

'But it's immoral to throw away good food!' Judi protests.

I remember somehow acquiring that view, too; but when we think about it realistically, it is clearly not relevant to our situation. For it cannot help any starving people if we eat up the left-overs. They are still starving, and we are getting fatter.

Certainly, better planning or reusing left-overs in another recipe might be a more moral reaction – and you will be less fat. Also, any money saved could be donated to a worthy cause.

**'So Demanding . . .'** The last part of the lament of the Patter of Tiny Feet goes: '. . . and she's so demanding that I'm exhausted and fed up and so I eat to cheer myself up and to give me more energy!'

Judi's right about one thing. Young children are very demanding and can exhaust a mum or dad who's looking after them. But what the carer needs is not the biscuits and chocs that she/he might fancy, but nourishing food to give sustained energy. Nutritionists now recommend that the best suppliers of those sustained levels of energy are the complex carbohydrates, such as wholemeal bread, potatoes in their jackets, high fibre cereal, wholewheat rice and pasta (but *not* accompanied by high fat products such as butter, margarine, cream, mayonnaise, oils). Also, a one-a-day multi-vitamin and mineral tablet will ensure that vital nutrients are not missed. Not so interesting as a choc bar, but it was energy you wanted, wasn't it? A fast boost of energy, provided by a high-sugar product like a chocolate bar, may be needed if you are doing a marathon or competing in a long bicycle race, but not for looking after children.

So much for energy. What of being 'fed up'? Maybe you are over-conscientious about amusing your child every minute of the day. Children need to learn to play independently and amuse themselves, and also must learn that they cannot expect mum (or anyone else) to gratify all their demands for attention immediately.

Help your children towards independence by giving them pictures to draw by themselves, puzzles to persevere with, blocks and models to build and work out by themselves. Encourage their independent efforts; prompt with words such as: 'try again', 'have another go', 'think about it', 'try something else', 'keep going', 'you're doing well', 'do some more', 'do it again', 'do another'.

Be generous with your praise when something has been made or done independently; a half-hearted 'Yes, that's nice dear,' is not so encouraging as phrases such as: 'that's a wonderful effort.' 'It's a beautiful picture, and you have worked so well on it by yourself . . .' 'You're getting very independent, that's great.' 'I love all the colours you've put on it, and so much work you've done.' 'You have worked a long time on that, fantastic!'

Assist your child's social development and your own sanity by joining with other mums and toddlers, or 'swap' by caring for each other's children regularly, while you have a nice time doing something that you enjoy − something other than eat! We are all entitled to pleasure and time to ourselves, of course, and there is no reason to hang on to the feelings of guilt that society seems to dump on to us.

## COUNTERACT WITH THINK SLIM
- Think Slim, realistically: 'it cannot help the starving millions if left-over food goes into my mouth. It won't help the starving millions but it will help me to get fat.'
- Treat yourself to complex carbohydrate foods, not instant energy, high-sugar snacks that will dump you in an energy trough soon after.
- Join forces with other mums to share child care and for company outside the home.

## 3 THE WORKING MOTHER JUGGLE
Perhaps you are performing the Working Mother Juggle? You hop, skip and juggle through your life: surviving the nine to five (or longer hours), doing the Supermarket Sprint, collecting the dry cleaning, whisking the duster, cleaning the loo, preparing the babyfood, rustling up a little something quick in the kitchen; and weighing yourself down with pangs of guilt about missing your baby's first word and worrying whether baby will ever grow up normally without a full-time parent − *and* you are trying to lose weight, too.

(I realise that some sole Fathers, too, are performing this circus act. Merely for convenience I shall use the term 'mother', but the comments apply equally to men in similar positions.)

I was a 'working' mum and wife, too, in the days when it was rare, and the not-so-Civil Service allowed me four weeks off before my baby's birth, and four weeks after. My only alternative was to resign under their policy of once resigned, never re-instated. I was pragmatic; I worked. So, I well know the stresses, particularly when lively baby doesn't like to waste a minute of this new life and wakes up frequently in the night.

However, even Working Mother Jugglers can succeed at losing excess weight, and they particularly need to Think Slim to do it. Some of the previous section 'At home all day with . . .' may apply to you too, so you could start by checking through that.

Next, parents who work need to be particularly organised. That may seem obvious, yet even people who are organised at their work-place do not always transfer this attitude to their home-life.

Dave was a single parent (after his wife left), looking after three boys aged ten, eight and two. He explains: 'It might seem odd, but even though my work was in project management in the computer industry, at first I didn't make the connection between managing things at work and at home.'

For some women the problem may be that they play the haphazard housewife because that is the 'little woman' role they have been conditioned into, and it does not prompt them to be efficient. The 'Little Woman' secretly fears that an efficient woman may be an unattractive one, threatening to her mate.

Have none of this nonsensical notion. If you are efficiently organised, slim and fit, you have both the time and energy to cement your relationship with your other half. Ensure, too, that your other half is just that, half of a relationship, having equal responsibilities as well as equal rights. If the other half does not share the chores equally, insist she/he does. Talk through who shall do what, and stick to it. Do *not* give in! (This applies equally with growing children, for they need to learn how to live and take responsibility for themselves in a family setting. Check whether you are actually training your children to be selfish, uncaring and exploitative, and if so, resolve to change that, now.)

A woman can allow her partner or family to be selfishly lazy over chores because it makes her feel needed. She is unconsciously trying to quieten her primitive fear of being abandoned by her mate and family, by making herself indispensable. Unfortunately, it doesn't work. No one can ensure that they will not be abandoned. It is a fear we have to live with, and remind ourselves that we are capable of surviving even if the 'worst' were to happen. Besides, there are millions of other potential mates out in the big wide world. So, avoid making your Working Mother Juggle even more difficult by playing 'Being Mrs Goodwife' (and read more about that trap in the 'Negative Wizards in Yourself' Section).

Finally, children can become your slimming allies. Talk to them about your slimming, encourage them to be considerate in buying you suitable presents.

Pam told me: 'My two children, Philip and Sara, who are 8 and 6, bought me low-fat yoghurts and a slimming magazine, all beautifully wrapped, for Mother's Day. I was delighted!' She has also lost 3 stones/ 19 kilos in weight.

## COUNTERACT WITH THINK SLIM
- Think Efficiency: live by lists.

- List your week, your month; your jobs/appointments.
- Prioritise your 'to do' lists.
- Take 15 minutes every morning to plan what must be done; a few minutes every evening to check that it has been completed.
- Take short cuts in food preparation, always Thinking Slim on calories.
- If home arrival time is slimming danger-time for you, when you nibble at baby's food or children's tea, make it a new habit to have only a drink for yourself, or a piece of fruit.
- Insist that partners are partners in chores, and that children take responsibility too.
- Ensure that you get enough rest, and do some relaxation.
- Refuse to try to Do-It-All.

## OVERCOMING OBSTACLES: PRE-MENSTRUAL SYNDROME

'For a few days before my period I just have to have sweet things to eat!' moaned Kay in exasperation. 'I don't know what comes over me!'

What 'comes over' Kay (and perhaps you too?) may be the effects of the Pre-Menstrual Syndrome (or PMS). This used to be called PMT or Pre-Menstrual Tension, but it has been realised that there are additional features besides tension, so it is now usually referred to as a 'syndrome', that is, a cluster of symptoms.

These symptoms occur and continue for two to fourteen days before a period and disappear as the period begins. They can be grouped into four main areas, which are:

1 The tension group: anxiety, irritability, tension, headaches, feeling unable to cope, tearfulness, clumsiness.
2 Food cravings, for carbohydrates or sweet foods.
3 Water retention (breast swelling and tenderness, bloating of the stomach and ankles). This results in weight gain.
4 Depression, lethargy.

Some women also report constipation during this time of the month.

Women generally do not suffer all of these symptoms, nor get them every month. PMS is more common in women who are over 30 years old, than in younger women.

What causes PMS? It is thought that as a woman's body goes through its monthly cycle of producing the female hormones that enable her to become pregnant, mainly oestrogen and progesterone, there can be an imbalance between the two which results in the symptoms.

If you wonder whether or not you are suffering from PMS, keep a Symptom Diary for three months; a suggested outline is presented on page 163. Mark in the types of symptoms in the 'code' suggested (or one of your own). You could keep more detailed comments in a Journal to help you to pinpoint the problems and find ways of alleviating or surviving them.

## PMS SABOTEURS OF YOUR SLIMMING:
## 1 THE TENSION FEELINGS

'I get so irritable, I could scream!' admits Anna.

'I bitch at people,' explains Jani.

'I could just burst into tears at the slightest thing!' agrees Kris.

'I get so clumsy. I drop things and make a mess and then get so cross with myself!' declares Emma.

All of these slimmers are suffering from aspects of the tension group of PMS symptoms; the slimming danger is that the very real tension is then alleviated by eating extra food.

## COUNTERACT WITH THINK SLIM

Try these general measures to alleviate PMS:

- Try taking a tablet supplement of 35 mg of the B6 vitamin, twice a day, and ensure the B group of vitamins are present in the multi-vitamin/mineral tablet you take each day. (Do not exceed 80 mg of B6 supplement as any excess has been suspected of causing damage to the nervous system.)

- There are other Vitamin tablets specially formulated to alleviate PMS syndrome, which include Magnesium. In Britain these are: 'Magnesium OK' and 'Premence', which are available over the counter at chemist shops.

- Evening Primrose Oil (in capsule form) has been known to help some women (but it is expensive to buy).

- Your low-fat, low sugar eating style as suggested in this book is exactly what is recommended by nutritionists to alleviate PMS. Cut out chocolate and sugar treats totally at this time.

- If you smoke, kick the habit.

- Reduce alcohol to none or minimum levels during PMS days, because it has a greater effect on the body at this time.

- Cut out caffeine: in tea, coffee, cola, chocolate.

- Forgive yourself any clumsiness. Accept it as part of PMS; allow yourself more time to do your chores at this time of the month. (You are already avoiding the 'Be Perfick' syndrome, aren't you? If not, read the 'Negative Wizards in Our Culture' section on 'Oughta-be Perfick', page 62.)

- Think Slim: remind yourself that there are ways of surviving tension and irritability other than by eating. Exercise is a very very effective one, as well as speeding your slimming. Also, be kinder to yourself during this time: re-schedule your workload; pamper yourself with baths, or even a visit to a Beauty shop (with the money you've been saving all month on snacks you've given up); have pleasant chats with friends or partner; rest and read; do some yoga, meditation, or relaxation.

- If tension plagues you, catch those tense thoughts ('I could scream!' 'Nothing seems worth it!' etc) and Stop them. Replace them with more realistic thoughts, such as 'I know this is only that old PMS again – I'll feel better soon!' and maybe think of nicer times to come.

- Fight any constipation by doing all of these three things:
  1 Eat high-fibre foods (wholemeal bread, cereal, jacket potato, fruit especially oranges and prunes, vegetables, beans and pulses).
  2 Drink enough fluids (3 pints per day).
  3 Take daily exercise (walking, swimming, cycling).

**Self-Help – Not Enough Help?** If the self-help measures suggested here produce no appreciable improvement after you have tried them seriously and consistently for a three-month trial, including keeping your record chart, you could consult your doctor and/or one of the organisations which advise women specifically and/or individually on PMS problems. (See page 274.)

## 2  THE FOOD CRAVING:

'I just have to have sweet things to eat!' was Kay's lament. This craving seems to be for carbohydrates. Usually we interpret it as a cry for choc bars rather than for a slice of bread, and the results can be very damaging to our slimming. The craving is real, but it is our interpretation that is astray. The body wants 'complex' carbohydrate, such as bread, cereal or potato, the only sort that were around in the early civilisations that Mother Nature originally placed us. But we think biscuits or chocolate. Both of these do contain carbohydrate, but they are basically 'refined' carbohydrates, with lots of sugar and calories, and, of course, very pleasant to eat. However, you won't use your craving as an excuse to indulge your desires, while kidding yourself that it's not your responsibility, will you? If you do, you will put on weight and fool no one but yourself. Tough, but true.

To alleviate the physiological craving, ensure that every three hours or so, some small amount of complex carbohydrate is eaten, such as a slice of bread or a low-cal crispbread or two. Time your meals to coincide with this three-hour feeding programme if possible; if not, keep to the complex carbohydrate snack each third hour. Taking food in this situation is similar to taking a medicine. If a doctor prescribed medicine for a cough, you wouldn't substitute a sweet milkshake and expect good results, so give your body what it needs, not the choc and bickies that you're lusting after. (Of course, you *can* have the choc and bickie lifestyle, but the price is being fat and being responsible for it.)

## COUNTERACT WITH THINK SLIM

- If your body craves carbohydrate, think what it needs: complex not refined carbohydrates, that is, bread/crispbread not biscuits/chocolate.
- Every three hours, eat a small portion of complex carbohydrate. Eat it *without* a fat spread, either dry or with one of the following: a smattering of marmite, half a banana, tomato and cucumber, very

little of a very low-fat cheese spread, or 1 oz/28 g of cottage cheese.

## 3  WATER RETENTION

'Every month I get "the boob job",' 'complains Sandi, 'and I put on weight on the scales.' Sandi regularly suffers from PMS water retention that causes swollen, tender breasts and a bloated tummy, and which is displayed on the weighing scales too.

During this time it's possible to gain 3–5 pounds/1½–2 kilos on the scales, and many slimmers, when they see this, discourage themselves with their frustrating thoughts: 'This isn't worth it! What's the use of trying to slim when the weight goes on like this?'

Then, to what do they turn to comfort themselves? A game of badminton? Fat Chance. A packet of 'elastic' biscuits (one is always followed by another because they are connected by invisible elastic) or some cake or ice cream. So 3 pounds of water retention soon becomes 7 pounds of fat.

## COUNTERACT WITH THINK SLIM

First, there are general measures which may help:

- Cut out added salt in your cooking and on the table, because salt encourages water retention. This may seem difficult at first, but it's very possible if you decide you *will* change. I did it 'cold turkey' in ten days, after which added salt became no longer part of my life. Alternatively, you can buy a salt substitute. (Ask at the chemist/ pharmacy: 'Lo-salt' is available in Britain, in Boots chemist shops.)
- Cut down on any processed food that is salty or has salt added to it, such as tinned ham or other meat, nuts etc.
- Caffeine can make water retention. Cut out caffeine in tea, coffee and cola. There are good caffeine-free alternatives. You're not wrinkling your nose already and thinking 'I don't think I'll like it!', are you? If so, read the Negative Wizard section on 'The Ostrich Position' (see page 71) and change your thinking. If you've tried one caffeine-free drink and don't like it, try another brand, and persevere. Anything which tastes different takes a while to get used to. Look for a solution, not another excuse. Chocolate also contains caffeine, so cutting that out for the PMS days may also help.
- It is not helpful to cut down on your total intake of (low-cal) liquid. Your body needs 3 pints/1·7 litres per day to function properly, and anyway, if you do restrict it, the body may simply hold on just as fiercely to its reduced amount.
- Some women find that over-the-counter or herbal diuretics help to shed some of the problem. (Diuretics are substances which increase the flow of urine.)

Then, if those measures don't help, there is the essential Think Slim:

- Sandi knows how to think; she is a realistic Think Slimmer by now, having lost over two stones despite such monthly miseries. She thinks, and says: 'Well, you just have to accept it; you know what it is, so you just carry on and don't let yourself get put off.'

- Such Think Slim needs to become a thinking habit. It is reminiscent of that very useful alcoholics prayer, to accept 'that which cannot be changed'. Re-read Sandi's words, and write them on a Think Slim card. Learn them off by heart.
- Say to yourself: 'It's only . . . pounds/kilos of water. I'm not going to make it into pounds/kilos of fat by my eating!'
- A Think Slimmer does *not* get obsessed with what the scales show.

## 4 DEPRESSION

'Just before my period I feel so depressed and wretched. Everything seems too much effort, and life just doesn't seem worth living,' mused Natalie. 'Then I think I'll have a bit of something nice to eat to cheer myself up . . . then another bit . . .'

'As well as feeling depressed, I just collapse into tears for no reason,' said Katie.

If depression plagues you, first you need to check whether it is connected to PMS or whether it's a separate message. Depression is often thought of as a visitation from heaven-knows-where come to torment us for no reason. In the past, doctors have often been quick to assume that depression is some form of mental illness or disturbance; yet it may be just that people are depressed simply because they live depressing lives.

The unorthodox psychiatrist R.D. Laing wrote about a woman whose husband took her to their GP because she 'felt like screaming'. The GP saw that she had a lovely husband, two delightful children, and plenty of money, and promptly sent her to a psychiatric hospital because he thought she must be mad. Or must she? Eventually, she was fortunate to be seen by Laing who was the first to ask her what it was about her life that caused her to feel like screaming.

Depression may be a symptom, a sign of an underlying dissatisfaction that you are not acknowledging – a scream that you are not screaming. Then the depression is a useful message to you that all is not well in your life. Useful, because if you can recognise what is bothering you, you can take steps to improve the situation.

If you are feeling depressed what is not well in your life? To help pinpoint underlying problems, try completing these sentences for yourself: 'I'm depressed about . . .' 'I'm depressed because . . .'

Or, depression may be a symptom of an underlying feeling of helplessness. Try completing: 'I feel helpless about . . .' and 'I feel helpless to change . . .'

Also, anger, unexpressed and turned inwards, can show as depression. Check this out by finishing the sentence: 'I'm angry about . . .'

Maybe the first time you try completing these sentences no relevant thoughts follow, but check a few times, particularly when you are fairly relaxed and have a few moments to yourself (in the bath?). Or, talk it over with a friend who can prompt you.

If you locate reasons within your lifestyle for your depression, set about thinking how you can change things. There is always a way, even though it may not be easy. Get help and support to do something positive, and you can swap your depression for action. Read the practical and wise book by Dorothy Rowe *Depression: the way out of your prison* or her more recent publication *Breaking the Bonds*.

While you are taking action, also follow the advice below to conquer your depressive thoughts.

If no reasons for your depression are apparent and you have kept your PMS Diary which indicates a cycle of depression connected to your period date, then your depression may simply be due to hormonal imbalances that are thought to cause PMS.

PMS RECORD CHART

| DATE: | MONTH 1 | MONTH 2 | MONTH 3 | SYMPTOMS KEY: |
|-------|---------|---------|---------|---------------|
| 1 | | | | A = Anxiety |
| 2 | | | | B = Breast tenderness |
| 3 | | | | C = Clumsiness (lack of |
| 4 | | | | co-ordination). |
| 5 | | | | Co = Constipation. |
| 6 | | | | D = Depression. |
| 7 | | | | F = Food cravings. |
| 8 | | | | L = Lethargy. |
| 9 | | | | M = Menstrual bleeding |
| 10 | | | | days. |
| 11 | | | | S = Swollen stomach. |
| 12 | | | | T = Tension (including |
| 13 | | | | irritability). |
| 14 | | | | |
| 15 | | | | |
| 16 | | | | |
| 17 | | | | |
| 18 | | | | |
| 19 | | | | |
| 20 | | | | |
| 21 | | | | |
| 22 | | | | |
| 23 | | | | |
| 24 | | | | |
| 25 | | | | |
| 26 | | | | |
| 27 | | | | |
| 28 | | | | |
| 29 | | | | |
| 30 | | | | |
| 31 | | | | |

## COUNTERACT WITH THINK SLIM

- Follow the nutrition and vitamin supplement guidelines for alleviating PMS already outlined.
- Catch those depressive thoughts ('I'm fed up!' 'Nothing seems worth it!' 'I can't be bothered', etc). Stop them. Replace them with more realistic and positive thoughts, such as: 'I know that this feeling is only due to that old PMS again. I'll feel better soon!' Or: 'I *can* be bothered!'
- *Do* something (except eat) so as to concentrate your mind on busy thoughts rather than depressive ones, or:
- Relax and fill up your mind with more pleasant thoughts, so there is no space for the depressions to haunt it. Think of fond memories or of nice times to come. If you don't have any nice future times planned, review your life, and plan some. They do not have to be extravagant events, maybe just some time out for yourself. If your family does not allow you time out, assertively insist on it. You deserve it, and need it. (Re-read the section on Assertiveness (page 26) to help you.)

# OVERCOMING OBSTACLES: NEW YEAR RESOLUTIONS

January 1st seems a good time to many people to start slimming to get rid of the festive flab, and to make New Year resolutions. So it is. However, the road to staying fat is, as we know, paved with good intentions and they are not enough.

Making resolutions is just like Target setting. You need to re-read Step 4 on targeting yourself before you make them.

Your resolutions need to be written down. You could increase your motivation by making them important-looking: sign and date them, hang them on your wall.

Set a date in your diary, or organiser, to review your resolutions. I set a monthly date with myself on the first Sunday of every month, at 11.45 am, when I check over my progress on my resolutions. That's an easy time for me to remember, and I do it, every month. It's surprising how well it works. Then, I add to my New Year resolutions by making mid-year resolutions, too.

If, on your review, you find you have slipped out of your resolved activity, don't shout at yourself and despair. Just check what got in the way, decide how to avoid that next month, and start again, resolving to do better (but not necessarily be perfect). This time, review yourself each week until your resolutions have been 'naturally' absorbed into your lifestyle. Just because you have slipped out of the resolutions – 'broken' them – does not mean that you should abandon them. Resolutions do not have to be seen as all-or-nothing things. Re-start them; adjust them; add to them.

Ginnie's resolution was to do 30 sit-up tummy-crunch exercises every morning. By the end of January she had missed about half the days; she would simply forget. So, she resolved to set a routine. She would always do the exercises immediately after her shower. Routine is very likely to help. It did. By April, Ginnie was doing her exercise every day, no problem, and her improved trim tight midriff was clear evidence. She was delighted. Less than two minutes invested every day had paid a great dividend. For you, the resolution does not have to be exercise. Choose your own; set a routine; review; adjust; start again after failure. By next year you will have succeeded.

# NOURISH YOURSELF!
## Think, eat, drink, be slim . . . and merry

Eat, drink and be Merry, for tomorrow we diet! Not any more.

What follows is *not* a Diet. If you were expecting to find a Diet, it would help you to go back to the beginning of this book and check out the ideas again. Sometimes what goes in one ear comes out the other (unlike calories, which go in one end and settle on the tum, waist and hips), especially if for you, while this book was in one hand, the hoover was in the other and the baby was screeching in your ear.

What follows are 'Nourish Yourself' eating guidelines and suggested menus that you can use for the rest of your slim-fit life.

However, the eating guidelines will only help you to become slim and stay slim if you also use the ideas and Think Slim strategies in the first five Steps.

## THE SELF-EMPOWERED SLIMMER THINKS AND CHOOSES

Every slimmer is unique, having a different lifestyle from any other slimmer. So, for any food and drink programme to be successful, it must be 'lifestyle-friendly' for many different styles of life. The only way that this is possible is for each slimmer to be the final designer of hishe/her own programme, working within given guidelines.

'I can get on with this slimming system,' confided Berenice, with a glass of Buck's Fizz in her hand. I had a glass of Buck's Fizz in my hand, too (but then in the fat old days I'd have had another and another and never compensated for the calories).

Berenice continued: 'I've been on diets before but they are so strict, I couldn't have had this' – she waves her fluted glass around expressively – 'so that I get to think life's hardly worth living. Then I give up the diet.'

Her husband approved of the Think Slim system, too. He smiled at me: 'So you're the one who's responsible for my new woman.'

'Not quite,' I responded, smiling back. 'Your wife is.'

So, the self-empowered slimmer takes responsibility for her/his slimming and employs 'thought for food'.

## THINK SLIM: THOUGHT FOR FOOD

She/he learns the guidelines (which follow) for:
- choosing foods
- preparing and cooking
- the portion amounts to eat
- how to eat

## THE THINK SLIM QUESTIONS

She/he thinks *before* eating:
   Do I really want this? No I don't. Shall I eat it? No I won't. Yes I do?
I'll make up for it, promise to.
   Is it worth its calories?

She/he thinks *while* eating:
   Am I really enjoying this?
   If the food's not fabulous, I don't waste the calories.
   If I don't want it, I don't have to eat it.

She/he thinks *after* finishing eating:
   Did I really enjoy that?
   Do I need to make up for those calories – and when and how shall I
do it?

## A LIFESTYLE FOR A LIFETIME

Think Slim is not about dieting; it is about learning a new style of slim-
fit eating and living which you can practise – and *enjoy* – forever.

   Psychology studies confirm what we know from our own experiences,
that mankind is a pleasure-seeking animal. There is nothing wrong with
that. Throw away any Puritanical religious ideas to the contrary.
Pleasure is fine as long as it is in moderation and with concern for the
rights of others.

   So, it would be nonsense to expect real human beings to deprive
themselves totally of their favourite foodie treats forever. Therefore, the
Think Slim Food and Drink Programme is designed so that you can
choose to include – *in moderation* – the favourite foods that many diet-
systems forbid.

   'Oooh, I think I can live with this . . .' enthused Bebe, in some surprise,
after her first three weeks, steadily losing weight, on the Programme.
That, of course, is exactly the idea.

   Nor does it seem reasonable to ban alcohol completely while you are
aiming for your desired weight. However, if you wish to speed up the
rate of your weight loss (still at a healthy rate) then you could choose to
give up your alcohol for a period of time that you choose. This would
certainly speed up your rate of losing excess weight. It's your choice. If
you wish to include alcohol, read the part of this Step: 'Cheers! Alcohol

Matters', before you finally decide on your strategy, see page 182.

## HOW TO THINK SLIM AND INCLUDE 'A LITTLE OF WHAT YOU FANCY'

Remember that the most important word in that phrase is 'little'. Moderation, with calculation, is the key.

Calculate the amount of your 'little' as follows.

- If you have over 2 stones/13 kilos to lose, allow up to 400 calories per day.
- If you have between 1 stone and 2 stones/6 to 13 kilos to lose, allow up to 200 calories per day.
- If you have under 1 stone/6 kilos to lose allow up to 100 calories only, twice per week – having them at the weekend is a good idea.

If you choose extras that are low in fat you will speed your weight loss.

**The week/weekend strategy.** Many slimmers have found it helpful to have a stringent slimming effort from Monday to Friday each week, with very few or none of the extra unit treats, and then include their extras only at the weekend. This system works well because it maximises the speed of weight loss while still allowing favourite food and drink treats; it is easier to say NO to yourself during the week when you know you are going to say YES to yourself very soon, at the coming weekend. Many slimmers find the weekend is the weaker end of their slimming, as social events and a lazier lifestyle encourage more food and drink; so don't fight it – build it into your slimming strategies. This system presents you with a routine eating and drinking habit that you can continue, keeping slim and fit, for a lifetime.

Experiment with finding the system that works best for you and fits best into your lifestyle; every slimmer is unique. Remember to reduce your extras as you have less and less weight to lose. Or, increase your exercise: see Step 7 'Move Yourself', page 199.

# NUTRITION MATTERS!

There is no point in being slim if you are not fit, healthy and full of vitality to really enjoy your slim life!

Our body is not just a designer appendage. It is more like a machine (think of it as like a car) which needs to be well fuelled and serviced to give its maximum performance. The 'performance' in this case is your life. It's the only one you've got, so to enjoy it more you need to look after your body more. Nutrition studies can guide us to feed our body in a balanced way to give it the fuel it needs to run at its best. So, nutrition matters.

However, you need not be any expert nutritionist. The British government has kindly done our homework for us. Nutrition and medical experts during the 1980s produced healthy guidelines for eating in the NACNE and COMA Reports. These have both been updated by the latest Report issued by the government in July 1991. This keeps to the same principles as those of the 1980s, which may disappoint those who love to stay stuck in their old eating habits with the excuse that 'the experts keep on changing their minds'. The guidelines are to:

- Cut fat, especially saturated fats such as butter and meat.
- Increase fibre – from fruit, vegetables and cereals.
- Cut refined sugar to not more than 12 teaspoons each day inclusive of all the hidden sugar in processed foods (such as tinned ham or beans, tomato and other sauces; chocolate treats – a Mars bar contains the equivalent of five teaspoons of sugar; and drinks such as cola which contains eight teaspoons per can).
- Cut salt.

The good news is that what's healthy is also suitable for slimming, and those expert guidelines are the ones we adopt in the Think Slim Food and Drink Programme:

| | |
|---|---|
| LESS FAT | MORE FIBRE |
| LESS SALT | MORE COMPLEX CARBOHYDRATES |
| MINIMUM REFINED SUGAR | MEDIUM PROTEIN |

If you understand the reasons for the guidelines, you are more likely to be keener to use them and to make wise choices – those that feed not fatten your body – so brief explanations follow here.

## 1 YOUR BODY NEEDS PROTEIN – IN MODERATION

Protein builds and repairs essential body cells, the very basis of your body. In children it is also essential for growth. It is needed daily.

Protein builds muscle – but no, it won't make you look like Rambo. Muscle means strength, and is needed for your body to move and carry things, like food!

There is one muscle of vital importance to your body: your heart. Most people don't think of it as a muscle, but it is, and it needs protein. Without enough protein, it may be damaged, and heart trouble/attack could result. This is a very real and potential danger from Very Low-calorie Diets (usually the liquid type) or any 'diet' which restricts daily calories to 500 calories or below (and therefore has too little protein).

It is thought that a woman needs about 2 ounces/50 grammes of protein per day. A man needs more, 3–3.5 ounces/75–90 grammes, if his job or lifestyle is physically active and/or he is over 6 feet tall. There is no need to try to 'count' your protein, if you follow the amount guidelines in the Eating programme.

**Good low-fat protein foods**: Lean meat, poultry, white fish, egg-whites, soya products, cottage/low-fat cheese and low-fat yoghurt.

**Other (less rich) protein foods**: Bread, cereal, rice, potatoes, pulses.

## 2  YOUR BODY NEEDS MORE CARBOHYDRATES – COMPLEX AND FIBRE

Carbohydrates come in three forms: Complex (starch), Fibre, Sugar.

### A  COMPLEX CARBOHYDRATES

Complex carbo's give you less-fattening filling power and energy for making the most of your life.

**Main complex carbohydrate foods**: Potato, bread, pasta, rice, cereals and beans.

### B  FIBRE

Think 'big-F'; fibre is a friend to your body and to your slimming. Once referred to as 'roughage', fibre is an indigestible carbohydrate which simply passes through the digestive tract helping it to do its job properly, to prevent constipation, and reduce the risk of bowel problems and cancer. Bowel cancer is common in the western world where we eat much less fibre than in the east, where bowel cancer is almost unknown. Bowel cancer is the third biggest killer in Britain, and usually goes undetected for too long. Reduce your risk by increasing the fibre in your eating programme.

Fibre is also a friend to slimmers because when it is accompanied by plenty of low-calorie liquid (three pints per day), it helps to give you that stomach-full feeling, so you are free from hunger pangs. The recommended amount of fibre per day is approximately 1 ounce/20–30 grammes.

**Main high-fibre foods**: Bran cereals and muesli (no added sugar), brown rice, wholewheat pasta, jacket potatoes, lightly cooked or raw vegetables, pulses, fruit.

### C  SUGARS

Sugars come in two types: 'The one you love' or refined sugar, and 'The one you don't care about' – naturally occurring sugar.

**Refined sugar**. The Bad News: your body does not need refined sugar (sucrose). Adam and Eve were not designed as customers for sugar factories (complaints to the Maker, please, not to me). Caveman and woman survived without boiled sweets and biscuits growing on trees. A certain choc bar, advertised to help you work, rest and play, may do so only in moderation, and with the realisation that you are eating for pleasure not 'need'.

Brown sugar is no healthier than white. Whatever colour, refined sugar is all empty calories. Empty Calories = Large Curves. More Empty Calories = Enormous Curves.

**Naturally Occurring sugar.** This is the sort of sugar that babies are born with a taste for. It is the naturally occurring sweetness of lactose in milk, or fructose in fruit.

Our inborn preference for natural sugars gets bastardised when mummies, daddies, grannies, Uncles Tom Cobley (and all) push western refined sugars into our baby food, and push sweeties, biccies and choccies into our tiny fists. We learn to have a very sweet tooth and a lifelong lust for high-sugar snacks that, ever after, plague our efforts to be slim.

Think-slimmers need to re-train their conditioned baby-habits back towards their natural-born taste for the sweetness of fruit.

'But I'm not as keen on fruit as I am on chocolate!' complained Gemma. I know how she feels. Nor am I. But if we continue to eat lots of refined sugar, we will never be keen on fruit. It is the excess sugar in our foods that makes us think that fruit has little sweetness. Eating less refined sugar does eventually re-educate the sweet tooth to less demanding proportions. At one time I, too, poured sugar on raspberries, complaining that they weren't sweet enough. Yet nowadays raspberries seem delicious in their naked state. It's my re-trained less-sweet tooth that's different, of course, not the raspberries. So, we can change our tastes with our habits.

Don't be fooled into buying a packet of 'fructose' to use instead of refined table sugar, believing that it is less fattening. Yes, it is 'sweeter' so that you may need to use less, but the calorie-savings are not high, and you are avoiding that important re-education of your taste.

## 3 YOUR BODY NEEDS LESS FAT

Don't dash for the biscuits! There are three types of fats/oils: saturated, poly-unsaturated, and mono-unsaturated. Just to complicate the issue, ALL fats contain a mixture of all three, so they are labelled according to which type is predominant.

### A SATURATED FATS

Your taste buds may like it, but your body does not need saturated fat. Worse, those regular fried bacon sandwiches may be storing up cholesterol in your arteries that can lead to a heart attack. Saturated fat is predominant in dairy products: butter, cheese, full-fat milk, yoghurt and cream; in margarines and lard and hard fats; in egg yolks; in meat (especially red meat).

Minimise your eating of these saturated-fat foods. Remember that even though fat may not be visible on your plate, it lurks, 'hidden' in some items such as chocolate, biscuits, cake, pastry, and ice cream. It can be too easy to forget that these are high-fat foods too.

## B POLY-UNSATURATED FATS
There are two 'essential fatty acids' in the poly-unsaturateds which are, as their name suggests, essential to your body's well being, and cannot be produced by it. However, you need very little; check that any oils you buy are labelled 'Poly-unsaturated' and use them sparingly.

## C MONO-UNSATURATED FATS
These are present in olive oil, nuts and seeds, and can be eaten health-wise, in preference to saturates. However, they are high-calorie items that slimmers need in very small quantities, if at all.

## 4 YOUR BODY NEEDS LESS SALT
In many modern foods, salt is flagrantly added (crisps and nuts) or hidden in the processing (tinned meats and packaged meals) and it is unlikely that you will suffer a shortage. So, don't add salt liberally to your cooking or to your plate. Salt can exacerbate high blood pressure, and water retention (sufferers of PMS please note!).

When you give up added salt completely, as I did, you get a wonderful surprise. Different foods actually have different and distinctive tastes. Mushrooms were my greatest discovery; they taste like mushrooms (instead of salt), and they are delicious.

It took me about ten days to become accustomed to food without salt. Yes, the first few days were agonising, but it gets easier.

## 5 YOUR BODY NEEDS VITAMINS AND MINERALS
The body system is rather like a jigsaw, with every piece playing an important part in the whole. Vitamins and minerals help the body to process the other food you eat. They are needed to complete the feeding of your body, and for your brain to function properly.

It is no surprise that people on very low-calorie crash diets (either liquid, or any mad-fad restrictive regime) can't concentrate to get their sums to add up, whether they be household accounts or company finances. For, the brain needs food too and often. Such diets don't provide all the vitamins and minerals needed by the brain.

So, a balanced wide range of foods is needed to ensure the full range of vitamins and minerals. I know that we are always being told by certain experts that if we eat a balanced diet we should get all the vitamins and minerals we need, but I am a realist. If you are slimming and if you are human (well, are you really prepared to choose some spinach every day?), and if you are getting your food from 20th century shops not the bottom of your organic garden, and if you boil your vegetables, then it is highly *un*likely that you will, every day, get the whole range of enough vitamins and minerals from your food. Some vitamins cannot be stored and are needed to be taken in *every* day (the B group, C, and folic acid).

The body's supply of vitamins and minerals is also plagued by alcohol, which depletes the body of these vital bits and pieces.

So, I believe that it's a helpful idea to take a one-a-day vitamin and mineral supplement. Check that the one you buy has minerals as well as vitamins. Women can benefit from included iron, although some women find that it doesn't suit them and prompts constipation; try one for yourself. It can be harmful to take more than the stated dosage; it is not true that if a little does you good, a lot will do even better.

Calories Count. Compare the calories that lurk in the same amount of different types of foods. It demonstrates that healthy eating guidelines are also slimming guidelines. Add the healthy eating guidelines to the slimming guidelines and you will get both slimness and fitness.

> PROTEIN: 3½ oz/100 g = 400 calories
> CARBOHYDRATES: 3½ oz/100 g = 400 calories
> FAT: 3½ oz/100 g = 900 calories

NB Protein foods often contain considerable amounts of fat, whereas complex carbohydrates do not; so, although their calorie count is the same, the 'health-fitness' value of carbohydrates is better.

## QUICK CHECK: THINK SLIM EATING STYLE
Reduce fat, increase fibre and complex carbohydrates.

Complex carbohydrates and high fibre foods will fill rather than fatten you. These are:

Wholemeal bread
High-fibre crispbreads
Potatoes in jackets
Brown rice
Wholewheat pasta
High-fibre cereals (no added sugar)

Oatmeal
Pulses: Lentils, dried peas, beans
Fresh fruit
Dried fruit
Vegetables

Also eat: low-fat foods.

Poultry
White fish
Shellfish
Low-fat cottage cheese
Low-fat cheese spreads
Quark

Fromage frais
Skimmed milk
Tofu
Low-fat yoghurt
Sorbets
Meringues

Eat, less often, in moderation: Medium-fat foods.

Lean meat
Low-fat burgers
Low-fat sausages
Low-fat minced beef
Oily fish (mackerel,
  salmon, sardines, pilchards)
Eggs (the yolk
  contains the fat)

Low-fat spread
Low-fat hard cheese
Semi-skimmed milk
Whole milk yoghurt
Greek strained
  yoghurt
Ice-cream

Eat only occasionally in small amounts: high-fat foods.

Red meat
Fatty meat
Fatty bacon
Butter
Cream
Margarine
Oils
Sausages
Pastries

Pies
Nuts
Chocolate
Sweets
Creamy desserts
Cakes and buns
Fried foods
Creamy/rich sauces

# ARE YOU GETTING ENOUGH?

Liquids, that is. Non alcoholic. Many people do not give their body enough to drink.

'But I'm not thirsty!' Debbie protests.

'But your body is!' I respond.

Often we remain unaware of the body's desire for liquid, or we mistakenly interpret the body's request for liquid as hunger. The body demands a drink, and we make it eat cake.

The body needs enough fluids to function properly. Strange as it may seem, we are made up mostly of water! On average, 70 per cent of a baby's weight is water; a woman's may be 40–50 per cent and a man's 60 per cent. Two thirds of the water is within our cells. The other third travels round our body in blood or other body fluids, or rests between cells as a 'cushion'.

Our body gets water from the water we drink, and the water contained in the food that we eat. It is also formed by our body's complex processes.

## WHEN IS ENOUGH ENOUGH?

On average, we need a *minimum* of 3 pints /1.7 litres of water each day for our body to function properly.

This could come from:

Drinks: 1¾ pints/1 litre

Food: ¾ pint/425 ml
Metabolism of food: ½ pint/285 ml

But, if our food intake is less than average, because of slimming, more of that liquid must come from drinks. Also, if we exercise, water is lost through sweating, and by breathing more intensely, so a drink after exercising is helpful.

Do extra drinks mean we put on extra fat? No, it is extra calories that add extra weight. High-cal drinks might make you fat; low-cal drinks help your body work well. If you drink more water than your body needs, any excess will flush through the body system. It will not settle as fat! Any excess will simply send you to the loo more often. The more water you drink, the more your urine will be diluted, and that's helpful, for concentrated urine may exacerbate problems such as kidney stones and cystitis.

Your body loses water all the time, by evaporation from the skin and lungs, and in the form of urine and faeces. A normal person may lose water as follows:

1 pint through the lungs
1 pint through the skin
¼ pint in faeces
2½ pints as urine

This makes a total of 4¾ pints per day! (The actual figure will vary between individuals.)

## CAFFEINE

Caffeine is an artificial stimulant that can be addictive and may prompt cravings for more, as well as feelings of irritability and even headaches. Who needs it?

Also unfortunate is that the quick boost in energy provided by caffeine is counteracted by a later energy 'dip'. That lethargy may then prompt the unwary slimmer to turn to a food snack to restore her energy level. So, caffeine is best avoided as far as possible. If you are accustomed to lots of caffeine, you may suffer withdrawal symptoms if you suddenly stop taking it; so it may be better to reduce your intake each day.

Strongly brewed coffee can contain 150 mg of caffeine per cup; instant coffee, 90 mg. A cup of tea contains 65–75 mg, and a can of cola about 40–60 mg. All can be bought in de-caffeinated form.

De-caffeinated products vary in taste just as do regular coffees and teas. So you may need to find, by trial and error, the brand of de-caffeinated that you prefer.

## NOT GETTING ENOUGH – THE PROBLEMS

If your body fluid drops below its required level, you will feel weak and lethargic. There is, simply, not enough water for your body to function at its maximum efficiency.

When slimmers feel weak and lethargic, they are likely, due to habit and lack of knowledge, to turn to food to 'give them some energy'. It isn't food the thirsty body needs – it's a low-cal drink. A reviving cuppa can revive a thirsty, weary body.

## THINK SLIM DRINK STRATEGIES
- Resolve now to check how much you drink, and ensure it is enough.
- Remember that alcohol dehydrates the body, so if you take some alcohol, you need to take more water/liquid to compensate.
- If you need to 'train' yourself to drink more (useful) liquid:
  - think of a 'Low-cal Drinking Plan' to suit your day's timetable
  - make yourself a schedule, a 'Drinks Diary', similar to the one which follows
  - carry your Drinks Diary with you, and complete it as you take your planned drinks
  - if you are at home all day, you can pour out your 3 pints/1.7 litres (or more) of water into a jug each morning, and use it all day to make hot drinks or cold.

## ARE YOU GETTING ENOUGH?

DRINKS DIARY (NON-ALCOHOLIC, LOW CALORIE)

NAME: .................................. DATE: ................................

|      | Morning | Afternoon | Evening | TOTAL |
|------|---------|-----------|---------|-------|
| MON  | ............ | ............ | ............ | ............ |
| TUES | ............ | ............ | ............ | ............ |
| WED  | ............ | ............ | ............ | ............ |
| THUR | ............ | ............ | ............ | ............ |
| FRI  | ............ | ............ | ............ | ............ |
| SAT  | ............ | ............ | ............ | ............ |
| SUN  | ............ | ............ | ............ | ............ |

# THINK SLIM COOKING PRINCIPLES
The food you choose may be reasonably low in calories, but it is important that your methods of preparing and cooking do not multiply those calories to sabotage your slimming. So, it's essential to Think Slim when you cook.

Having a slimmer in the family need not mean separate cooking. For the healthy cooking guidelines that are good for slimmers are good for the family too.

Men can benefit from such an eating style, not only to reduce a paunch, but by obtaining some protection against premature heart disease to which they are particularly vulnerable.

Children can benefit from making slim-fit eating a lifelong habit, thus avoiding our problems. So, for them, the earlier the better. Babies should be fed on the newer no-added-sugar baby foods wherever possible. Young children should not be given confectionery as snacks – use fresh fruit instead. Buy a variety, including 'exotic' ones like kiwi, mango and Sharon fruit.

Give love – not sweets. Many parents who want to give love make the mistake of giving sweets instead. When you want to give love, give a cuddle, or loving words. Or a non-food treat. Share your time, talk, play a game.

Child-favourite foods like beefburgers, fish fingers, beans and chips can continue. Make sure that the products you use are of best, low-fat, quality. Perhaps make your own beefburgers, solely with low-fat minced beef – it's quick and easy. Buy low-sugar baked beans, use microwave or oven chips, and wean on to baked potatoes as often as possible. I know a mum who refuses to fry chips, ostensibly because of the mess and smell in the kitchen, and has successfully weaned all her family onto baked potatoes.

Remember that making a child fat does him/her no favours!

The cook can use the Think Slim cooking guidelines, for all the family, without drawing attention to them. The taste can still be great! Think Slim cooking means thinking about both preparation and cooking of food.

## PREPARATION
- Cut off all visible fat from meat
- Remove all skin from poultry/game *before* cooking
- Weigh (not guess) your portions
- Scrub instead of peeling potatoes and other vegetables – many vital nutrients are contained just below the skin
- Don't nibble or taste as you prepare

## COOKING
- Best methods: Dry-fry (in a non-stick pan), grill, poach, steam, bake, pressure-cook.
- Avoid fat-frying: no oil, lard, butter or margarine. If a recipe tells you to pre-fry ingredients in butter, simply miss this stage out. Or, if you prefer, you could use two teaspoons of a poly-unsaturated cooking oil (eg sunflower, rapeseed) or olive oil.
- Avoid roasting, except very occasionally.
- Dry-fry minced beef first, then drain off the fat and discard, before

continuing.

- Avoid deep-fried chips, except occasionally; then cut chips straight and chunky (not crinkly and thin) so that they will absorb less fat. Alternatives to deep-fried chips are shallow frying, or pre-packs suitable for grilling, oven-baking or microwaving.
- Avoid thickener in casseroles. Instead, when almost cooked, drain off the liquid, and boil it rapidly to reduce and thicken it instead.
- Don't nibble or taste as you cook. If you must taste a new recipe, one teaspoon is enough, rather than a tablespoon.

## SUBSTITUTE LOW-CAL LOW-FAT ALTERNATIVES WHEREVER POSSIBLE

- Substitute skimmed milk instead of whole milk in drinks, sauces, custard, and milk puddings. Also, use to mash potatoes, and scramble eggs.
- Substitute a 'fatless' sponge for a 'Victoria' cake recipe.
- Substitute low-fat, no-added-sugar yoghurt, with fresh fruit, as a filling in a sponge cake, rather than cream and jam.
- Substitute low-fat, no-added-sugar yoghurt for cream in casseroles, where possible. (But don't then allow it to boil, or the yoghurt will curdle.)
- Substitute low-cal alternatives for cream.
- Substitute sorbet, or yoghurt ice-cream, or low-fat ice-cream for Cornish or rich varieties. Use it to accompany a sweet, or fruit pie, instead of cream or custard.
- Substitute wholemeal rice and pasta for white. It's more filling.
- Substitute wholemeal flour for white, or use half and half.
- Substitute low-fat spread for butter or margarine on bread, crispbread etc.
- Substitute jacket potatoes for chips and boiled potatoes.
- Substitute low-fat roast potatoes for traditional ones; use larger chunks, brushed lightly with oil, cooked in a non-stick tin.

# ENTERTAINING

All of the Think Slim cooking guidelines can be applied when you are entertaining. Your guests will not be aware of your Think Slim cooking – they will only be aware of the great taste.

Discard your old conditioning – don't think you are obliged to slave over a hot stove all day to be an acceptable host/hostess. Many supermarkets sell wonderful food 'boxes' which you can use as a basis for any or all of your courses at your dinner parties. If an appreciative guest asks you for the recipe, you can choose whether to be honest ('I dallied with a packet'), or enigmatic ('it's an old family secret'). Of course, if you enjoy cooking for guests and have the time available, carry on. It's your life and your choice.

Make presentation a priority, not only of the food, but of the table setting too – and of your slimmer self. Choosing a cold starter and/or a cold sweet, minimises your cooking and presenting problems.

Good slim-fit 'starters' include melon balls with purple grapes in port; prawn cocktail (low-cal dressing); prawns on pink grapefruit; smoked salmon with low-fat cottage cheese; crudités with low-cal dips; low-fat pâté.

Good slim-fit cold desserts include fruit salad; fruit on meringue; low-cal trifle; low-cal cheesecake; sorbets; sundaes mixed with low-fat ice-cream and yoghurt; fresh fruit and low-fat cream substitute; fruit fool made with yoghurt and no added sugar.

Whether you are cooking for the family, or entertaining, remember that you don't have to discard your favourite cookery books. Simply think again about your recipes, operating the guidelines above. You can also treat yourself to the newer 'low-fat, slimline' cookery books. For suggestions, see the Further Reading section, page 275.

Finally, avoid The Ostrich Position ('I don't think I'll like it') when faced with new recipe ideas. Train yourself to unaccustomed flavours with small tasters. Experiment with herbs and spices. Don't bore yourself with repetitive, or dull food. Meals can be delicious as well as nutritious and slimline.

## CALORIES COUNT!

You don't have to total up *all* your calories with this Food and Drink programme. The suggested basic day will allow you 1000 calories, then you choose your add-on extras. However, it is extremely useful to know the approximate 'cost' of food in calorie terms. Cheap calorie counters can be bought at your newsagent or bookshop.

## THREE GOLDEN RULES OF CALORIE THINK SLIM

1 There is no such thing as a free lunch – especially for slimmers. Just as everything you buy in a shop has a price tag, everything you eat has a price tag, in calories rather than money. So, some foods are expensive and you need to decide if you can afford them, just as you would decide whether you can afford that beautiful little number on the hanger, or that super-sports in the showroom. Think: 'Can I afford it?'

The Think Slim Golden Rule No. 1 is: Is it worth its Calories? It's a principle that most of us budget-conscious folk use for our purchases, so it is simple enough to transfer it to food.

2 It can be easy for the unwary to gobble more calories than intended.

Carrie had discovered a new salad she'd bought and enjoyed with her lunch sandwich. 'Delicious,' she drooled, but she hadn't looked at the label to check the calories. It was salad, and salad is slimming food, isn't it? We checked the now-empty tub: 310 calories. She had eaten two at lunch-time as well as a sandwich.

The moral is the second Golden Rule of Calorie Think Slim: never put anything in your mouth unless you know how many calories it's got.

Nowadays, manufacturers are much more helpful with displaying the calorie count of their foods. Never go shopping without your reading glasses! Also, calorie-count booklets are readily available at newsagents for less than the price of three chocolate bars.

3 The third Golden Rule is: If it's not worth its calories, don't eat it! There is no point in being a masochist. We are looking for pleasure in our lives and in our food, and if it's not there, opt out.

James, out with his business colleagues, ordered his favourite lemon meringue pie for dessert. When he tried it, it tasted as if the lemon had never been anywhere near a lemon tree, and as if the meringue had never been related to a real hen. To the amazement of his colleagues, he threw down his cutlery and announced: 'That's not worth its calories!' and went on to the coffee. James was right. He was employing Think Slim. 'If the food's not fabulous, don't waste the calories!'

## CALORIES COUNT: THINK SLIM
- 'Is it worth its calories?' 'Can I afford it?'
- 'I don't put anything in my mouth until I know how many calories it's got.'
- 'If the food's not fabulous, don't waste the calories.'

## CHECK YOURSELF/TEACH YOURSELF:
Following is a Basic Calorie Count Quiz, for you to check out your knowledge, so that you know the 'price' of what you are eating. Knowing about calorie-costs will not guarantee your slimming success (many a Calorie Mastermind is still overweight, just as I once was), but without it you may make calorie mistakes that lead to your slimming failure.

| How many calories in? | Approx Calories |
| --- | --- |
| 1 oz/28 g butter | ............................. |
| 1 oz/28 g margarine | ............................. |
| 1 oz/28 g full-fat hard cheese | ............................. |
| 1 oz/28 g shortcrust pastry | ............................. |
| 1 oz/28 g wholemeal bread | ............................. |
| 2 oz/56 g potato (uncooked) | ............................. |
| 2 oz/56 g brown rice (uncooked) | ............................. |
| 2 oz/56 g wholewheat pasta (uncooked) | ............................. |
| 1 medium egg, white only | ............................. |
| 1 medium egg, yolk only | ............................. |

1 oz/28 g lean beef, when cooked ..........................

1 oz/28 g lean chicken, without skin, when cooked ..........................

1 oz/28 g chicken, including skin, when cooked ..........................

1 oz/28 g milk chocolate ..........................

Answers on page 265.

## 'THAT LI'L BIT WON'T HURT' – OR WILL IT?

An extra 50 calories a day adds:

350 calories each week
18,200 calories each year

18,200 extra calories each year can mean a weight gain of about 6 pounds/2½ kilos.

In five years 6 pounds/2½ kilos weight gain each year can mean a weight gain of 30 pounds/13½ kilos.

In ten years 6 pounds/2½ kilos weight gain each year can mean a weight gain of 60 pounds/27 kilos.

The extra 50 calories could be a nibble of cheese, a square of chocolate, half a cream biscuit, a tablespoon of tasted gravy, a lick of double cream, 10 grapes or 10 peanuts. Think slim: calories count.

## 'CHEERS!' ALCOHOL MATTERS

'Another little drink won't do you any harm,' they urge you. But is this really true, especially for the person who wants to be both slim and fit?

The wise slimmer is aiming not only to reduce excess weight, but also to remain fit and healthy. So, the reduced number of calories available need to be 'spent' wisely to give the best possible food value for the calories consumed.

Alcohol is quite high in calories, but it contains *no* nutrients, that is, it has no food value, so you cannot nourish yourself with alcohol. It is possible for a heavy drinker to be fat *and* suffering from malnutrition.

Alcohol is sometimes referred to as 'intoxicating liquor'. The word 'toxic' can remind us of alcohol's 'poisonous' effects on the body. The long-term effects of excess alcohol include liver damage (hepatitis and cirrhosis); cancer of the mouth, throat and gullet; stomach disorders such as ulcers, gastritis and bleeding; high blood pressure; brain damage; depression; and sexual difficulties. Short-term, alcohol promotes accidents, arguments, violence, and may lead to disruption of personal relationships.

## HOW MUCH IS TOO MUCH?

The British Health Education Authority recommended that the 'safe' health limits for alcohol are 21 units per week for men, and 14 units per week for women. (See page 65 regarding alcohol units.)

Slimmers may be affected by alcohol more than 'heartier' eaters because food intake is being restricted and therefore alcohol is absorbed faster by the digestion. It is not advisable to 'save' alcohol units and imbibe them in one or two sessions a week, for a sudden large intake is likely to be even more damaging to the body.

Additionally, alcohol impairs judgement – not only for driving, but for eating too. Many a slimmer, under the influence of alcohol, succumbs to the temptations of over-eating. Then, a hangover leads to miseries that may be consoled with biscuits and other comfort foods.

It may be best for the slimmer to exclude alcohol completely. However, alcohol has become very much a part of our modern culture and social lifestyle. So, an alternative is to reduce alcohol intake.

Think Slim and drink with the following tips:

- When you account for your calorie intake remember that 'home measures' are generally much larger than 'pub measures'. You can purchase a measure from good department stores, and if you wish to drink at home, regularly, you need to buy a measure and use it every time you pour.
- Remember that low-alcohol drinks are not necessarily low calorie. Check a calorie list.
- Avoid lunch-time drinking. Apart from its bad effects upon your afternoon functioning, the later drop in blood sugar levels will send you reaching for more alcohol – or extra food – later in the day.
- Plan alcohol-free days each week. Decide which days, and stick to them. Establishing a new habit makes success more likely than a vague resolve to 'cut down'. Or, restrict your (moderate) alcohol intake to the weekends.
- Pace your alcohol intake throughout the evening.
- Decline to get involved in buying 'rounds', if drinking in a group.
- 'Lengthen' your alcoholic drink with low-cal mixers or soda.
- Do not 'top up' your alcoholic drink with another (unless with soda or low-cal mixers). Finish each measure first, or you will not be able to count your intake.
- Say 'No' in a way that sounds like 'NO', rather than 'persuade me'.
- If saying No is difficult for you, try an assertiveness course or self-help book. (See 'Further Reading', page 275.)
- If you use alcohol to give you confidence in a social situation, acquire your confidence elsewhere. Again, an assertiveness class is useful, or a self-help book.
- Remember, you don't have to be a drinker to be a real man. Many women admire a man who can say 'No' to alcohol. Nor do you have to drink to appear sophisticated, whether you are a man or woman.

- If you are dependent upon alcohol, seek expert advice. (See 'Useful Addresses', page 273.)

## THE THINK SLIM SLIM-FIT FOOD AND DRINK PROGRAMME: PUTTING IT ALL TOGETHER

Suggested menus follow; but *first* please read these instructions.

This Food and Drink Programme is designed for adult women and men (over 18) who are, as far as they know, in good health and have no special medical dietary requirements. However, if your doctor requires you to be on a low-fat or low-cholesterol diet, this programme *is* suitable. You should take this book to your doctor (show this page), to check hishe/her advice. The programme is based on high-fibre, low-fat, medium protein, low-sugar, low-salt principles.

### INSTRUCTIONS

- Take a one-a-day vitamin and mineral tablet each morning.
- A basic day's menu is made up of your choice of:
  One breakfast
  PLUS one sandwich/packed lunch/light meal
  PLUS one main meal
  PLUS 'a little of what you fancy' extras.
  You can eat them in any order.
- Also: have up to 1 pint/560 ml of skimmed milk (or 2 low-calorie, low-fat yoghurts) per day.
- Note: drink 3 pints/1.7 litres of low-calorie fluid per day. This is *important* for your health, fitness and your slimming.

## SPECIAL CATEGORIES OF SLIMMERS

### MEN OVER 21 YEARS: SEDENTARY JOB/LIFESTYLE

Add to the basic day's Menu:
3 oz/85 g (3 thin slices) bread
3½ oz/100 g boiled/baked potato/rice/pasta
Extra 'free' vegetables as you wish
½ pint/285 ml skimmed milk

### MEN OVER 21 YEARS: PHYSICALLY ACTIVE JOB/LIFESTYLE

Double the amounts on the basic day's menu in respect of skimmed milk, potato, bread, pasta, rice, vegetables, fruit.

Increase by half, the amounts of white meat and fish.
Keep red meat to the same amounts as shown.

### YOUNG ADULTS 18–21 YEARS

These are generally still 'growing' years, and your body needs more good

food. Add to the basic day's menu:
  Young men: 4 oz/110 g (4 thin slices) bread
  3½ oz/100 g boiled/baked potato/rice/pasta
  Extra 'free' vegetables as you wish
  Young women: 1 oz/28 g (1 thin slice) bread
  More 'free' vegetables.

## WOMEN OVER 40 YEARS
You may need to restrict your extra 'little fancies' as, unfortunately, the metabolic rate (the rate at which energy is burned up by the body) has a tendency to decrease with age. 100 calories daily may need to be deducted from the 'little of what you fancy' guidelines. You need to experiment. You could also counteract this annoying natural tendency by increasing your exercise. Refer to Step 7 'Move Yourself' (page 199) for ideas.

## SLIM-FIT DAILY CALORIES
The Basic Day of suggested menus gives you approx 1000 calories each day; then you calculate your extra 'little fancies'.
   You can vary the menus by planning them yourself to a 1000 calorie basis. Substitute calorie-counted low-fat recipes that you find in other publications. Choose poultry and white fish most often as a basis rather than red meat. Don't forget to add in items like gravy, and cook-in sauces.
   It is unhelpful to go below 1000 calories on a regular basis. Your body may simply adapt to exist on less calories and you will find it more difficult to lose weight and much easier to put it back on.
   If you have had extra in a celebration, refer to 'The Day After the Night Before Stringent Settler' on page 193–4.

## SPACING YOUR MEALS
Do have some breakfast. It does not have to be a large meal. Divide your breakfast and eat some of it later during the morning if you prefer. Breakfast is important because:
– your body is in need of food after fasting all night
– you will feel more alert and energetic, and less likely to fall into foodie temptation or 'low' moods that trigger binge eating
– you will avoid the 'must have a choc bar' physical craving at elevenses
– your metabolic rate will fire up after you have eaten breakfast, and burn off your calories quicker all morning.
   Space your meals *regularly* throughout the day. This is to give your body the regular fuel it needs to perform properly. Be kind to your body – it's the only one you've got. Spacing meals also avoids the binges that may be triggered during the evening due to 'starvation' days.

## PLANNING, SHOPPING, AND COOKING
All of these issues are dealt with separately in this book. However, a brief

summary is presented here for quick reference.
- Shop for high-fibre, low-fat, low-calorie substitute ingredients and packaged food.
- Prepare all food with high-fibre guidelines in mind, eg leave skins on potatoes, other vegetables and fruit, where possible.
- Cook all food according to low-fat cooking principles, as already explained (grill/steam/dry-fry/microwave).
- If you are cooking vegetables, lightly steam them, to avoid boiling away all the vitamins and minerals.

## BREAKFASTS:
Choose from:
1 oz/28 g of your chosen high-fibre muesli or cereal (preferably no added sugar)
ADD: milk from your allowance *or* a tub of low-fat yoghurt
                       *or* 1 chopped apple
                       *or* 1 small banana
                       *or* tinned fruit in natural juice


2 oz/56 g toast (check the weight of the bread)
2 *level* teaspoons low-sugar jam or marmalade. (LEVEL!)

2 oz/56 g toast (check the weight)
1 egg, boiled or poached

¼ pint/150 ml unsweetened orange juice. (Try diluting it with a little water.)
1 small egg, boiled or poached
2 crispbread *or* 1 oz/28 g toast

1 grilled rasher bacon
1 tomato
1oz/28 g mushrooms (boiled or heated without fat/oil)
1 small egg, boiled, poached or 'fried' in a non-stick pan without any fat, *or* 1 oz/28 g toast or bread

1 small tub low-fat yoghurt
PLUS: up to 3 pieces of fruit, chosen from apple, orange, pear, small banana or ½ banana

Breakfast Power Drink:
1 banana
⅓ pint/190 ml skimmed milk
2 egg whites
Optional: 1 teaspoon wheatgerm, sweetener to taste
Blend ingredients together into a drink. If you need an express start to

your morning, make it up the night before and leave it in the refrigerator. If you prefer a hot version, blend banana and milk together, then heat (do not boil), remove from heat and add whisked egg whites, optional wheatgerm and sweetener.

IMPORTANT NOTE: Do not add any butter, margarine, or low-fat spread to your bread or toast unless you count it out of your 'Little of what you fancy' daily allowance.

# SANDWICHES AND PACKED LUNCHES

2 oz/56 g bread (2 slices; if *you* cut it, weigh it!)
*or* 4 slices Nimble
*or* 4 crispbreads

ADD fillings, choose from:

Chopped egg (one, size 3) with low-cal salad cream, plus cress, lettuce, or sliced tomato.
2 oz/56 g prawns, with dessertspoon Waistline seafood dressing, or low-calorie mayonnaise.
2 oz/56 g cottage cheese; add a little onion, Branston pickle or piccalilli, or grained mustard.
1 oz/28 g grated low-fat cheese (Edam, Tendale or Shape); add tomato and onion or a *little* Branston pickle or piccalilli.
1½ oz/40 g tuna, (in brine, *not oil*!); add chopped onion and Waistline salad cream.
1 oz/28 g ham; add mustard.
1 oz/28 g mackerel (in brine, *not oil*!); add a little low-calorie salad cream.
1 oz/28 g cooked beef; a *little* horseradish sauce, or mustard.
2 oz/56 g cooked chicken; add a little low-calorie salad cream, and chopped onion.

Accompany with home-made coleslaw – see recipe following. Also have an apple, or one piece other fruit (small banana) or, low-calorie, low-fat yoghurt.

## EVE'S EXOCET COLESLAW RECIPE

This coleslaw is delicious, nutritious, filling – *and* low-calorie. Nicknamed 'Exocet', as it's been called the slimmer's secret weapon, this filler-food has made all the difference to slimmers who have suffered in the past from feeling hungry and lethargic on a diet.

Basic Ingredients: white cabbage and onion.
Chop, and add one or more of the following: Cucumber, Carrot, or Celery.

Dress with a low-calorie salad cream, or oil-free vinaigrette, or seafood dressing mixed with a few shakes of bottled lemon juice. Try it out – put in as much or as little onion as you like. My favourite is cabbage with lots of onion and cucumber. Also try:
Cabbage – Onion – Carrot
Cabbage – Onion – Carrot – Cucumber
Cabbage – Onion – Cucumber – Celery
Try the different dressings, to add variety.

You can quickly chop up enough for a few days; leave in the fridge, and put the dressing on when you are ready to use it.

Eat with your sandwiches, or as a salad: take it to work in a container.

## EXTRA VEGETABLES
These may be added to your Light and Main meals (which follow) in sensible quantities: raw, or cooked *without oil*: asparagus, aubergines, bean sprouts, broccoli, cabbage, carrots, cauliflower, celery, courgettes/zucchini, cucumber, green peppers/capsicum, lettuce, marrow, mushrooms, onions, runner beans, spinach, swedes, tomatoes, turnips. *Not peas or sweetcorn* – if you want to add these, you must count the calories from your 'Little of What You Fancy' extras.

# LIGHT MEALS

### BAKED BEANS ON TOAST
7.9 oz/225 g can Weightwatchers baked beans.
1 oz/30 g toast (no spread)
or use small tin of beans and 2 oz/60 g toast

### FILLED JACKET POTATO
5 oz/140 g potato, baked in jacket

CHOOSE FROM FILLINGS: 3 oz/85 g cottage cheese
1 oz/28 g grated low-fat cheese (Edam, Tendale or Shape), chopped onion, sliced tomato
2 oz/56 g prawns, 1 dessertspoon Waistline seafood dressing, or low-cal mayonnaise
Small tin Weightwatchers baked beans

### OMELET
2 small eggs (size 3)
Make omelet in non-stick pan *without* fat.
Fill with one of these fillings: 1 oz/28 g lean ham, chopped; 1 sliced tomato
2 oz/56 g mushrooms, cooked in water; ½ chopped boiled onion
1 rasher lean bacon, chopped; 1 sliced tomato

SOUP
1 packet Slim-Soup. Add *extra vegetables* if you wish
1 oz/28 g bread

BACON and TOMATO
1 rasher bacon, chopped
Sliced tomato, lightly cooked, no oil
2 oz/56 g mushrooms, cooked in water
1 oz/28 g bread

SCRAMBLED EGG ON TOAST
2 size 3 eggs, scrambled with skimmed milk
1 oz/28 g toast
*or* scramble one egg, and have 2 oz/56 g bread

TUNA ON TOAST
2 oz/56 g tuna in brine
2 oz/56 g toast

# MAIN MEALS

## AT YOUR CONVENIENCE: USING CONVENIENCE AND PRE-PACKED FOODS

FISH FINGERS
3 fish fingers, grilled
5 oz/140 g potatoes, boiled, jacket, or mashed with *skimmed* milk
3 oz/85 g peas

SHEPHERD'S PIE
8 oz/225 g Bird's Eye shepherd's pie
*or* own-made; *no* fat for cooking minced beef
Mashed potato with skimmed milk. (Serve 8 oz/225 g total weight)
3 oz/85 g peas *or* other *extra vegetables*

COD IN BATTER
1 Bird's Eye cod in wafer-light batter, grilled or 'fried' without fat
4 oz/110 g grill or oven chips
1 oz/28 g peas, and *extra vegetables*

LOWER-FAT BEEFBURGER
1 lower-fat beefburger, grilled or 'fried' without fat
4 oz/110 g grill or oven chips
1 oz/28 g peas, and *extra vegetables*

PIZZA
6 oz/170 g Findus French Bread Pizza *or* Lean Cuisine French Bread Pizza
(or other 'baby' size Pizza)
Vegetables or own-made Exocet Coleslaw (see recipe, page 187–8).

ANY *LEAN CUISINE* OR *MENU MASTER* OR *HEALTH CUISINE*
AS MAIN BASIS
You will find Cod in Sauce, Chilli, Lasagne, Spaghetti, Curry, Canelloni,
Oriental Rice. Add lots of extra vegetables and 3 oz/85 g potatoes.
(Sorry, no peas with these, unless out of your 'A Little of What You
Fancy' extra allowance.)

RICE MEALS (CHINESE AND CURRY)
1 Ross Stir-Fry pack, any flavour
'Fry' with 3 tablespoons water – no oil!
Add *extra vegetables* (not potatoes) if you want to

COOK IT YOURSELF
STEAK AND CHIPS
4 oz/110 g (raw weight) lean steak
4 oz/110 g grill or oven chips
1 grilled tomato
1 oz/28 g peas
(Mushrooms can be added if cooked *only* in a little water)

SUNDAY/ANY DAY ROAST
3 oz/85 g lean beef, lamb, pork, duck *or* 4 oz/110 g chicken (skin
removed)
2 roast potato pieces, to weigh 3 oz/85 g in total, *or* 6 oz/170 g jacket
*or* boiled potato
1 dessertspoon stuffing
2 tablespoons unthickened gravy (*or* 1 tablespoon thickened).
*Extra vegetables.*

LAMB OR PORK CHOP
5 oz/140 g lamb or pork chop, fat removed; grill or oven cook
6 oz/170 g potato, jacket/boiled (or 4 oz/110 g mashed, skimmed milk)
1 oz/28 g peas OR sweetcorn.
*Extra vegetables.*

COD IN SAUCE
5 oz/140 g cod
Make white sauce with skimmed milk, but no butter or margarine. Add
either cooked onion, mushrooms, or ½ oz/15 g grated lower-fat cheese
(Edam Tendale, or Shape)
6 oz/170 g baked potato, or 5 oz/140 g mashed with skimmed milk.
Chosen *extra vegetables.*

## CASSEROLE – CHICKEN OR LIVER
4 oz/110 g chicken or lamb's liver
½ small onion
chopped carrot
2 oz/56 g mushrooms
1 stock cube (optional)
Put in a casserole. Slice 4 oz/110 g potato thinly and place on top. Cook in oven for one hour (180°C/350°F/gas mark 4).

**Important note:** It is *vital* to weigh the amounts for your portions. When we guess, we *always* guess more – never less.

## EAT A LITTLE OF WHAT YOU FANCY
- If you have over 2 stones/13 kilos to lose, choose up to 400 calories each day.
- If you have between 1 and 2 stones/6 to 13 kilos to lose, choose up to 200 calories each day.
- If you have under 1 stone/6 kilos to lose, choose up to 100 calories *only* on two days of the week – the weekend?

| FRUITS | | CALORIES |
|---|---|---|
| Apple (5 oz/140 g) | | 50 |
| Banana (weighed with skin, 7 oz/200 g) | | 90 |
| Orange (peeled, 5 oz/140 g) | | 50 |
| Pear (5 oz/140 g) | | 50 |
| Raspberries (fresh, 3½ oz/100 g) | | 25 |
| Strawberries (fresh, 3½ oz/100 g) | | 25 |
| Grapes (3 oz/85 g) | | 50 |
| Plums, Victoria 1 | | 40 |
| Blackcurrants (stewed without sugar, 3½ oz/100 g) | | 25 |
| Gooseberries (stewed *with* sugar, 3½ oz/100 g) | | 50 |

| THE DEMON DRINK | | CALORIES |
|---|---|---|
| Beers, ½ pint | | 90 |
| Brandy, Gin, Vodka, Rum, Whisky (⅙ gill/25 ml) | | 50 |
| Wine (4 fl oz/110 ml) | sweet | 100 |
| | medium/dry | 75 |
| Sherry (⅓ gill/50 ml) | sweet | 70 |
| | medium | 60 |
| | dry | 60 |

## OTHER DRINKS

| | |
|---|---:|
| Orange juice, Britvic (4 fl oz/110 ml) | 50 |
| Grapefruit juice (4 fl oz/110 ml) | 50 |
| | |
| Milk, skimmed (½ pint/285 ml) | 100 |
| Milk, full-cream (½ pint/285 ml) | 200 |

## SWEET FOODS                                    CALORIES

Biscuits:
| | |
|---|---:|
| Digestive (1) | 75 |
| Digestive, chocolate (1) | 140 |
| Jaffa cake (1) | 50 |
| Gingernut (1) | 45 |

## CHOCOLATE                                      CALORIES

| | |
|---|---:|
| Milk chocolate bar (1 oz/28 g) | 150 |
| Kit-Kat (2-finger bar) | 110 |
| Mars bar (1) | 266 |
| Mars bar, fun size | 100 |
| Bounty bar | 266 |
| Wispa bar | 200 |

## MISCELLANEOUS                                  CALORIES

| | |
|---|---:|
| Jam (1 *level* teaspoon) | 25 |
| Meringue Nest (1) | 50 |
| Polo Mints (8 sweets) | 50 |
| Yoghurt (Eden Vale SHAPE) | 57 |

## FATS                                           CALORIES

| | |
|---|---:|
| Butter or margarine (1 oz/28 g) | 200 |
| Low-fat spread (1 oz/28 g) | 100 |
| Salad cream dressing (1 oz/28 g) | 90 |
| French dressing, Waistline oil-free (per tablespoon) | – |

## CARBOHYDRATES                                  CALORIES

| | |
|---|---:|
| Bread, wholemeal (1 oz/28 g) | 60 |
| Potato, boiled (1 oz/28 g) | 23 |
| Potato, roast (1 oz/28 g) | 45 |
| Potato, chipped | 75 |

| NUTS AND CRISPS | CALORIES |
|---|---|
| Peanuts, roasted and salted (1 oz/28 g) | 160 |
| Bombay-Mix (1 oz/28 g) | 140 |
| Crisps (1 oz/25 g pack) | 130 |
| Low-fat crisps | 120 |

*You can include other items of your own choice, as long as you count the calories.*

If your 'little of what you fancy' is made mainly of sugar or chocolate, it is a good idea to wait until the evening to eat it. For, if you eat sugary treats during the day, it is very likely that in a couple of hours you will be wanting some more. Then it will be hard to resist for the rest of the day and evening. Instead, if you eat them during the evening, hopefully by the time you are getting your follow-up craving, you will be in bed and asleep!

## THE DAY AFTER THE NIGHT BEFORE STRINGENT SETTLER

This is not a 'normal' day eating plan, but may be used for one day at a time after a day when you have eaten extra due to some celebration, etc. Do not follow for more than one day at a time.

BREAKFAST
1 low-cal yoghurt and 1 piece fruit
*or* 1 egg, poached or boiled

LUNCH
2 oz/56 g bread (*weigh it*) or 3 crispbreads. (Sorry, no spread)
1 oz/28 g ham (*weigh it*) with sliced tomato or cucumber
*or* 2 oz/56 g prawns with low-cal salad cream
*or* 2 oz/56 g cottage cheese, with tomato/cucumber
ALSO 4 oz/110 g Eve's Exocet Coleslaw (see recipe, page 187)
OR 1 low-cal yoghurt and 2 pieces fruit

AFTERNOON OR EVENING SNACK
1 apple or orange

DINNER
6 oz/170 g cod, in skimmed milk sauce
*or* 4 oz/110 g chicken, casseroled
OR Any low-cal ready-meal (eg Lean Cuisine/Menu Master)

*Add* Up to 6 oz/170 g any *extra vegetable* but no potatoes

Also drink plenty of low-cal drinks during the day

## THE THINK SLIM AND SLIM-FIT USEFUL SHOPPING LIST

You can adapt your shopping for yourself and the whole family will benefit, healthwise.

### CONVENIENCE FOODS

Convenience foods are not necessarily 'junk' foods. 'Good' convenience foods include:

Wholemeal bread, and 'ready-to-cook' French bread
Pitta/Lebanese bread
Frozen vegetables (which retain their vitamins and minerals)
Frozen fish (without batter or sauce) including prawns
Pre-packed mackerel, peppered; or with mustard
Fresh fruit
Dried fruit
Wholemeal bread
Wholemeal pasta (spaghetti, noodles, lasagne sheets, etc)
Brown rice
Dried beans
Dried pulses (lentils, peas, beans)
Low-fat calorie counted ready-to-cook meals

### CANNED FOODS

Tuna, and mackerel, in brine. Avoid if canned in oil.
Salmon (especially 'Keta')
Tomatoes
Tinned fruit in natural juice, or water
Low-sugar baked beans

'Poor' or 'junk' foods to beware of include processed and high-fat foods like made-up burgers, sausages, meat/pork pies, etc, where the proportion of saturated fat is likely to be high.

### CEREALS

Muesli base (a mix of cereals only, from health-food shops No fruit or nuts included. Add your own fresh fruit)
Any 'no-added-sugar' muesli
Kelloggs All-bran (although this does contain some added sugar)
Birds 'Grape Nuts' (stay crunchy in milk or juice)

### DRINKS

Decaffeinated coffee
Low-cal squashes, especially Wells Diet Orange (no added colouring)
Low-cal fizzies (including mixers for alcohol)

Mineral waters. Scottish Strathmore offers various 'hint of' flavours: lemon, lime and orange
Herbal teas

## SUBSTITUTES
Low-fat spread to replace butter/margarine (Lowest-Gold, Delight, Outline, Shape). Note that, generally, high-polyunsaturated margarines eg, Flora, are *not* low-calorie
Skimmed milk to replace full/half fat
Sweeteners: 'Canderel' Spoonful/Dispenser. No saccharine-type aftertaste, but do not add to boiling liquid – wait till it's off the boil.
      'Sweetex' Spoonful/Dispenser. Can be used for cooking.
Low-fat hard cheeses (eg Shape, Tendale, Delight)
Low-fat cheese spreads (eg Primula), portions (eg Delight) and processed slices (eg Weightwatchers by Heinz)
Low-fat pâté
Low-cal soups
Sugar-free jelly
Low-sugar jam
Low-cal salad cream (any make) and low-cal mayonnaise
Waistline low-cal oil-free dressing
Waistline low-cal vinaigrette dressing
Waistline low-cal seafood dressing
Kraft 'Continental Classics' reduced calorie vinaigrette

## ORGANISING YOUR SHOPPING
'It's when I'm shopping for food that I fall into temptation,' explains Gail.

If you, like Gail, nibble, surplus to requirements on your shopping trips, there are Think Slim strategies that can help you. However, apply your Think Slim Strategies even *before* you set off for the shops:

### BEFORE YOU SET OFF SHOPPING
- Plan a time to go shopping when you will not be hungry, to minimise the danger of a hunger-craving for food which you finally satisfy with too-handy, tempting, fattening snacks.
- Write out a shopping list – when you are not hungry.
- Take the shopping list with you – and stick to it.
- Take with you a low-cal snack, in case you are delayed and become hungry. (A crispbread, a piece of fruit, celery or carrot.)
- A flask/Thermos of ready-made tea or coffee could be taken with you, or left in your car, ready to quieten hunger pangs and impulsive eating.
- Carry powdered skimmed milk for drinks taken in a cafe, or in a friend's house. The powder can easily be carried in an empty tablet-bottle.

## WHEN SHOPPING

- Avoid passing the confectionery shelves if possible, or, adopt the 'blinkers' technique. Just like a highly strung racehorse wears blinkers so that he can only see forwards, to shield his eyes from those things that might startle him, you can adopt the 'eyes forward' approach to seek out only the shelves you need, avoiding the high-cal temptations. I used to yell silently to myself in sergeant major style: 'eyes forward!'; but now it is an easy, automatic style of shopping in food halls (but not in the frock shops, where my eyes are everywhere over the size 12s and below).
- Instruct your bossy demanding children to purchase their sugary treats for themselves, if possible. Don't buy sugary/fatty foods for very young children who have not yet learned how to be your boss. Buy fruit.
- Don't purchase 'Economy' packs of choc-sugar treats. You know there is no economy, merely temptation that you're not likely to resist before you get home.
- If your store does not stock the low-cal substitute foods that you want, tell (or write to) the manager.
- Read food labels. (It becomes quick with practice.)

## FOOD LABELS

By law, the label must show a complete list of ingredients, in descending order of weight. So, for example, if sugar appears highest on the list, it is proportionately highest among the ingredients. There is, so far in Britain, no law making other nutrition information compulsory; it is still being considered. But, a label may include information similar to this:

| NUTRITION INFORMATION | |
| --- | --- |
| Energy | 1212kj/289 kcal |
| Protein | 27.0 g |
| Carbohydrate | 14.4 g |
| Fat | 14.1 g |
| Sodium | 2.1 g |
| Fibre | 0.6 g |

Calories, per pack
Sometimes shown as 100 g:
check weight of pack.

'Carbohydrates' means starch *and* sugar. Refined sugar may or may not be shown separately. Sugar may appear as sucrose, fructose, or lactose.

Kilojoules are an alternative measure, (equal to × 4.2 calories) and can be ignored. Additives also appear on most labels, listed under their E-numbers.

Vague claims like 'all natural' may have no realistic meaning and may have large amounts of refined sugar and saturated fat.

Foods marked 'for diabetics' are not advantageous to slimmers. Although no sugar is included, its replacement is high in calories.

Do read labels. Don't be put off by jargon and figures. It becomes easier and quicker with practice and your slimming and fitness can benefit.


## HOW TO EAT

You don't think you need any advice? You're already an expert on how to eat? Just check out these tips.

**Eat slowly** – many overweight people are quick eaters. That does not mean that eating quickly makes you fat and that eating slowly will get you slim (unfortunately!). However, eating quickly often leaves you feeling less than full, for it takes time (maybe as long as 20 minutes) for the message that you are full to get from your stomach to your brain. So, when you eat quickly, you think the fatal words: 'I'm still hungry. That wasn't filling enough. What shall I eat next?' And you always find a calorific answer!

Also, if you are first at the dining table to finish, you feel a little envious of those still eating before your very eyes, and maybe you feel a little deprived. Then you are helping yourself to seconds before there's time to say 'huge hips'.

**Use a smaller plate for yourself.** You need to cut down on portions (of some foods) to slim, and using a smaller plate can help your brain to think that you've got as much as the bigger-eater next to you. Then you'll feel more satisfied.

**Sit down to eat.** Sitting down won't help the calories to disappear (unfortunately), but if you sit and concentrate on your eating, you get more pleasure from your food. The more pleasure you get, the lesser amount of food that you need; this is the 'more pleasure from less calories' principle. You feel more satisfied, psychologically, and are less likely to forage for more.

If you make a habit of eating on the hoof, you will already know how it feels to look around in astonishment and say, indignantly: 'Where's the rest of my sandwich gone?' You glare suspiciously at everyone from the spouse to the parrot, but eventually you realise that you must have eaten it yourself. But you didn't notice!

Food *is* there to be enjoyed. As slimmers, we need less food, so we want maximum enjoyment from it. Sit and savour every mouthful!

**Eating habits are precisely that – habits.** The power of habit means that if we do something twice, we are likely to repeat it. Do something rewarding (such as eating) 60 times or 600 times and we're hooked into 6 million times. So bad eating habits get a hold on our behaviour and on our bums, tums and legs.

Habit eating can be good-habit eating instead of bad. So, start new habits and think new Think Slim phrases:

'I don't eat in the car.'

'I don't buy chocolate or food treats with my newspaper or petrol.'

'I sit down and enjoy my food.'

'I eat slowly, and allow my stomach time to feel full.'

# MOVE YOURSELF!
## Exercise your imagination, and more

'I just can't imagine myself slim!' If you, like Jen, have been overweight for many years, perhaps it's difficult to imagine yourself slim. Yet it's important that you try to do just that.

Jen succeeded, at over 50, to become slimmer than she ever had been since her son was born, over thirty years ago. The length of time you have been overweight does not, as I have already pointed out, mean that it can't be done. The slimming laws of nature apply to everyone. But, even if you have been slim until quite recently, sometimes it can be difficult to imagine yourself back in those too-small clothes.

'I can hardly believe I used to get into that skirt!' said Tara incredulously. Yet she did, not so long ago, and she will again as long as she turns that thinking around: 'I used to get in that skirt so there's no reason why I shouldn't do so again.' If she *thinks* she can't, she won't make the efforts, and she won't succeed.

So, whether your excess weight is recent or long-standing, it is very helpful for you to exercise your imagination to help you see yourself slim. Also, our 'self-image' is like a picture held in our subconscious mind which we strive to keep. If that subconscious picture is a fat one, we might find some unconscious resistance entering our thoughts, working against our real desire to be slimmer.

## EXERCISING YOUR IMAGINATION
How to do it:

**1 Through any odd moments of day-dreaming.** Anytime you have a moment to day-dream, such as while waiting in a traffic jam, or a queue, use the wasted time profitably by day-dreaming of your slimmer self. Imagine yourself in various scenes: slipping into slimmer clothes, buying from the smaller-size clothes rails, getting into a smaller swimsuit and going to the beach or pool. Imagine people complimenting you on your slimmer shape, and see yourself smile happily and just saying 'thank you'.

**2 Through 'relaxation'.** By 'relaxation' I mean something very specific, and very different from simply being slumped in front of the television watching a favourite programme. I mean a state of proper relaxation of both your body and your mind, which you have deliberately set out to achieve. If you have already been to any relaxation or yoga classes, you will know what I mean, and will probably already be able to relax yourself. If not, you can learn how to do it by using instructions which follow.

Using your imagination, to see yourself as slim, or to imagine yourself confidently dealing wisely with eating situations, can be even more effective if you do it while in a state of relaxation. This is because we are thought to be more receptive to ideas and learning when our brain is relaxed, working at a slower level with deeper, relaxed 'alpha' brain waves. It is now believed that the left and right sides of the brain have different functions. The left side of the brain is believed to deal with the rational, pragmatic aspects of thought. The right side is the intuitive, creative side, maybe encompassing the 'unconscious' part of our mind that Freud suggested could have great, yet hidden influence on our everyday behaviour. It is this side that may be more easily tapped into, during periods of relaxation.

## HOW TO RELAX YOURSELF

Choose a time and place where you are likely to be undisturbed and where you feel comfortable, for up to about 20 minutes; and where you have a reasonably comfortable easy-chair (preferably with arms) or a carpeted floor that you can lie on. (Your bed may not be the best choice, for it may well be too comfortable and you will simply fall off to sleep. Do *not* try this sort of relaxation if you are in the bath, nor while driving a car.)

If you have less than 20 minutes to spare, it is still worth doing the relaxation. You would benefit from as little as three minutes.

If it is important that you spend no longer than 20 minutes, set your watch, clock, or timer to alert you after 20 minutes (in case you drift off to sleep) while you are first getting used to re-alerting yourself.

Otherwise, notice the time you are beginning, and notice the time you wish to finish. As you begin to settle down, tell yourself: 'I shall relax for twenty minutes until . . . time, and then wake up.' Repeat this to yourself again, before you begin. You will find that this should be enough, with practice, for you to alert yourself, and you will soon not need any alarm system.

If you lie down, try to lie in a position with your knees bent up and your feet flat, apart about the width of your hips. This position gives the best support for your back. Just experiment with the position until you are comfortable and your knees can relax without falling either inwards or outwards.

Your arms relax by your sides, palms facing upwards. Keep your head comfortably supported by the floor or chair but don't throw back your head.

## SEQUENCE FOR RELAXING:

1 Tighten up your hands into a fist, and tighten your arms. Keep them tight, tight, tight (say it to yourself three times, once per second). Relax them, palms upwards.

2 Tighten up your feet and legs. Keep them tight, tight, tight (say it to yourself three times, once per second). Relax them.

3 Tighten up the middle of your body. Keep it tight, tight, tight (say it to yourself three times, once per second). Relax it.

4 Tighten up your shoulders. Keep them tight, tight, tight (say it to yourself three times, once per second). Relax them.

5 Tighten up your face; screw up your features. Keep them tight, tight, tight (say it to yourself three times, once per second). Relax them.

6 Swallow, and leave your mouth just slightly open, to keep the tension away from your jaw. If, at any time, you feel a little tense, swallow again, and remember to allow the mouth to stay slightly open.

7 Take a nice, deep breath, in through your mouth and out through your nose. And another. Settle down nicely, enjoying the feeling of relaxation.

Now start to use your imagination to see yourself slim, and to see yourself slimming successfully.

See yourself slim, imagine yourself where you live, in your room, walking around, slim and fit, going about your daily life.

Imagine yourself standing on your scales, weighing yourself. Notice the weight on the scales stop at the weight you (wisely) want to be; feel comfortable and pleased with that.

Imagine yourself going into a clothes shop and going to the slim size clothes rails. Take a smaller-sized garment, try it on and see how it fits. Look in a mirror, feeling good and confident about your slim self.

Imagine yourself going somewhere special, perhaps to a celebration or a party. Imagine yourself going as your slim self; imagine your clothes; imagine someone paying you a compliment, feel happy and confident, smile back and say 'thank you'. Feel good as your slim self.

Think of other scenes for yourself, from your own life.

You can also use your imagination, in this way, to strengthen your motivation, by imagining yourself saying 'No thank you' to people tempting you to high-cal foods that you don't want. You could rehearse difficult situations that you may have to face.

You could simply repeat some of your Think Slim Prompt Cards, such as the simple: 'I am absolutely determined to slim' which will help you to keep your determination high.

Repeating other Think Slim Prompts, such as, 'Is it Worth Its Calories?' helps to fix the thoughts in your mind so that you use them at the appropriate time.

You could choose some from the checklist of Think Slim Prompts, 'An Eschatological Think Slim List', which appears on page 265.

Or, you could tape record your own instructions onto a cassette tape for your own use, if you think it would be helpful to you to start your relaxing session off. Also, see page 257 for details of a special Think Slim audio cassette.

## EXERCISE YOUR BODY – WHY BOTHER?

At one time the only thing I ever exercised was my imagination, usually thinking about what I could eat next. From being the Girl Most Unlikely, I now exercise regularly – not because I love it – but because I have been convinced of the benefits.

I hear many a new slimmer protest: 'Exercise? I'm always on the go – I never stop!' Well, that's better than sitting at a desk all day, but for optimal slim-fitness, 'on the go' is not enough.

My first realisation that exercise was a boon to slimmers was on a weekend away in a hotel that had a gymnasium and swimming pool. I used the gym, and in particular the exercise bike, and found at the end of the food-indulgent weekend that I had put on no weight! I was thrilled. Exercise suddenly seemed like a good friend! It is.

I used to think that people who exercised were some strange, different breed of fanatical humanity that had nothing in common with me. Then I found out that I was wrong, for I noticed other people who inspired me. My then boss at work went jogging each lunch hour, and explained that he did it, not because he was a jog-fan, but so that he could indulge more in the food he loved without getting fat.

Soon after, I was comparing notes with another male colleague who worked at keeping himself fit – also not because he loved it, but because of its benefits. I was then rather proud of myself because I was doing my tummy-crunch exercises daily – eight of them. He did them, too, he said. He was 51 years old, and slim.

'How many do you do?' I asked, curiously.

'Fifty to sixty,' he replied, in a matter-of-fact way.

I was flabbergasted, both at his total number and his matter-of-fact accepting attitude, and I determined that my measly eight would increase. I decided on 30 to 40, and that's what I do now. It takes less than two minutes each morning.

Since then, I've met women and men who swim 30, 40, 60 lengths and consider it all a normal part of the day's work; men and women who cycle a hundred miles a week; women and men who get on their exercise bike for 30 minutes a day (and a woman who does the 'odd hour' every day), and they all have two things in common. They're slim-fit and they do it not because they are exercise fanatics, but simply because they want the benefits. They do it without moaning or fussing; they do it because they have accepted what has become a fundamental Think Slim principle: 'There's no such thing as a calorie free lunch' or 'Nothing Achieved in Life is Achieved Free'. I admire them, and decided to join them.

## EXERCISE: THE SLIM-FIT BENEFITS

It is possible to become slim without exercise. But becoming slim-fit is a better aim, and achieving it is faster and more effective with exercise. Why? Obviously, exercise uses up calories, but it is now thought that there are additional benefits.

1 Your basic metabolic rate (BMR) is thought to be speeded up; an effect that lasts, so that after the exercise session, extra calories continue to be used up. This is the 'slim while you sleep' effect.

2 Muscle develops. The body becomes more shapely, with less flab.

3 A muscle-developed body burns up more calories than a flabby body of the same weight.

4 Exercise lifts the spirits, by causing the brain to release mood-lifting hormones, your own natural anti-depressants.

5 Exercise increases your physical fitness so that, overall, you have more energy and stamina. You are less likely to feel tired and so start prowling for a pick-me-up-biscuit.

6 Your body becomes more supple which makes general movement easier, so that you are less likely to suffer from strains (which cause miseries that are consoled by comfort eating).

7 Exercise is a good stress-reliever, whether you are a harassed business person or harassed child-carer, so you are less likely to start the stress-slide towards the sponge cake.

8 Aerobic exercise (explained later), three to four times per week, is thought to act as a preventer of premature heart disease. Men, if you wish to survive the 'dangerous years' between the ages of 40 and 55, please note.

9 While you are exercising, you are not eating.

What else do we want from an exercise programme? 'I've not much time for exercise!' warns many a busy slimmer. Nor have I. We both want an exercise programme that can be fitted reasonably into a Real Life. This programme assumes that you are a busy real person rather than a professional fitness freak who can spend hours on work-outs. It also assumes that you've read the first five steps to Slim-fitness in this book, are Thinking Slim so won't make excuses, and that you will make some changes to your time-table to fit in exercise.

## WHAT SORT OF EXERCISE?

Most 'experts' advise you to find a method of exercise that you enjoy. Fine if you can find any. What about the rest of us? I'm afraid that my Think Slim Exercise Advice is tougher, more realistic – and it works:

1 Think what we want to achieve and think which forms of exercise will achieve it.

2 Choose from those forms of exercise (where possible) a method of exercise that, to you, is the least of the evils.

3 Decide to do your exercise programme simply because of its benefits.

4 Build exercise – *as a routine* – into your lifestyle.
5 Accept exercise as a part of your life.
6 Don't moan about your exercise programme.

**1 What we want to achieve from exercise.** Think Slim is a holistic approach. It recognises that people are whole beings: neither just a mind, nor just a body. Think Slim is about empowering the person through the mind, and about empowering the body, too. Empowered for what?

The Thinking Slimmer basically wants a body that is slim enough and fit enough to really enjoy life; that is, a powerful body. I call it Think Slim BodyPower.

Some people begin exercise unthinkingly, never defining what they want. So, many men do weight training, even though they never need to lift heavy weights in their daily life. They achieve a muscular body (and if that is something they want, fine), but they are not able to run for a bus, or with the dog, for they have not bothered to strengthen their heart. So, even though they look 'fit', they may be prone to premature heart collapse. Squash fanatics are liable to drop dead on or off court if they do not strengthen their cardio-vascular system to cope with the severe bursts of stress that squash can put on their untrained hearts. On the other hand, joggers may have a fit heart but be crippled by muscle strains and injury; so can the go-for-the-burn aerobic dancers whose 'jumping jacks' jar and injure their joints, knees and ankles. Some slim women have their slimness spoiled by thick middles and slack midriff, tum and leg muscles.

So, the Think Slim BodyPower Programme is well thought-out to minimise injury and maximise slim-fitness and a toned shape, while still allowing you some choices.

**2 Choose from those forms of exercise (where possible) a method of exercise that, to you, is the least of the evils.** It is over-idealistic to think that there is a form of exercise out there that every one of us will love, if only we look far enough for it. A dedicated comfort-lover like me would be looking (and getting fatter) forever. Think realistically.

The largest proportion of exercise needs to be aerobic, and within that you can make choices. If you absolutely hate one type of exercise, choose another (that you merely dislike!). Don't get into the Ostrich position ('I don't think I'll like it') or you will doom yourself to not liking it.

Try. Persevere. Don't say: 'I tried exercise once and it didn't suit me.' Maybe you'll get to feel neutral about it, or even enjoy some of it. Maybe not. Consider the next point:

**3 Decide to do your exercise programme simply because of its benefits.** 'Yes but, it's Boring on a bike!' slimmers sometimes protest, starting to play the 'yes, but' game.

Think rationally. Separate out those things that you do for pleasure from those that you do for their benefits. Exercise, like cleaning your teeth and having a wash, is for benefits. If you enjoy it, that's a bonus.

Indeed, an exercise bike is not boring if you read while cycling. A good magazine or book can keep me (and you) pedalling happily. Stella recently reported how she did five minutes extra before realising it, because her magazine was so interesting. I, too, have been known to do minutes extra to finish an un-put-downable-book. It is the only time that I allow myself to read novels or light reading, so that I actually have something to look forward to on the bike. Otherwise you could watch television, or listen to the radio.

Think benefits. Give up to get. Give up your time and effort to get slim-fit, because the benefits are worth it. Life's too short to live it fat.

Fundamental Think Slim: Make efforts not excuses.

**4 Build exercise – *as a routine* – into your lifestyle.** I get on my exercise bike each morning for at least twenty minutes, as a matter of routine. Never do I ask myself 'shall I get on the bike today?' – because I know that my natural lazy tendency might tempt me to answer 'I'll not bother'. Now, the exercise bike is as normal a part of my daily routine as is cleaning my teeth. Just as I never ponder whether or not to clean my teeth, nor do I wonder whether or not to exercise. I just do it.

This 'lifestyle routine' works. Other slimmers have successfully copied it. Carole says: 'I just do it every morning. And I really feel more awake afterwards. I feel better than I ever did when I just went straight to work.' Carol has kept her target weight for over a year now.

There is also another benefit that Carol mentions: hard exercise followed by a shower makes you feel alive, alert and vital.

Of course, for you, exercise doesn't have to be in the morning. It's your life – set your own routine. Just don't play the 'No time' game (read the Negative Wizard Section 'No time' to re-educate your thinking).

**5 Accept exercise as part of your life.** Exercising, getting up earlier, changing your routine – it's all a matter of how you think about it. One of my slimmers, Dot, inspired me. She gets up at 5 am, is at work by 6 am and doesn't finish till 4 pm. I used my Think Slim: 'If she can do it, so can I.' So can you.

Accept. That means accept the necessity of exercise in your thoughts, your words and by doing it. Don't ask yourself 'shall I today?' Just do it. Also, repeat, often, to yourself and anyone else who cares to listen 'yes, I exercise . . . every day on my bike . . .' (or whatever you do).

**6 Don't moan about your exercise programme.** Moaners make them-selves, and everyone around them, miserable. Why think thoughts that will make you feel miserable? Don't 'awfulise'. Keep your thoughts in proportion. I know I'd prefer to do my cardio-calorie time on my exercise bike reading my thrillers than, cave-person-like, racing after an antelope to kill for my meal; or be washing by hand, carrying coal and suffering unwanted pregnancies as did my great-grandmother.

# THE BODYPOWER PROGRAMME

My notion of BodyPower is inspired by the lion and the lioness: they are lean, lithe and magnificent. They have power, pride (self-respect) – and a smile on the corner of their mouth.

### BodyPower: Three Aims, Three Methods

| AIM = | LEAN | LITHE | MAGNIFICENT |
|-------|------|-------|-------------|
| Method | Fat-burning, minimum-injury, maximum-power aerobic exercise | Body movement exercises | Body toning and tightening exercises |

Such exercise can give you that good-to-be-alive feeling that sends a smile to the corner of your mouth, as does being slim and fit; as do the things you do when you are slim, fit and self-empowered.

## 1 BECOMING LEAN

Being lean is about lacking body fat. Exercise that best helps us to become lean is that which burns up lots of calories in a relatively short time. It can achieve another aim, too: strengthening the heart so that as you go about your daily life, your heart can work less hard and can cope better with any emergency demands put upon it.

The exercise we need to achieve this slim-fitness is aerobic.

### AEROBIC EXERCISE

Aerobic means, literally, 'with air'. Aerobic exercise raises the rate at which your heart beats, the rate at which your muscles burn energy and therefore the rate at which we burn calories.

Examples of aerobic exercise follow. (Four stars equal best value; one star equals least value.)

| | |
|---|---|
| **** | Brisk walking (with vigorous arm-swings). Outside, or on an electric treadmill machine |
| **** | Exercise-bicycling |
| **/*** | Cycling |
| ***/*** | Low-impact aerobic exercise classes (dance; step) |
| */**/*** | Low-impact aerobic exercise video tape |
| *** | Swimming |
| *** | Aqua-aerobics |
| * | Jogging |
| * | Running |
| * | Rowing |
| * | Skiing |

If, in that list, you can spot a form of exercise that you already enjoy, great. Otherwise, join me and choose one that you dislike least and that you can fit into your lifestyle least inconveniently. Also, one that minimises your chances of injury and maximises the aerobic value.

It's your choice; but please consider the following plus and minus points before deciding:

| | | |
|---|---|---|
| **Brisk Walking:** | + | Minimises injury; must be brisk, not a stroll. |
| | ? | Will you go out in all weathers? (Or find an alternative form of aerobic exercise?) |

| | | |
|---|---|---|
| **Electric Treadmill:** | + | Use as an at-home, all-weather 'brisk walking' machine, if you can afford to buy one. The non-electric types don't seem very satisfactory to most users. |

| | | |
|---|---|---|
| **Exercise Bike:** | + | Minimises injury. |
| | + | Can be done in comfort at home. |
| | + | Easy to monitor progress with milometer, etc, on the bike. |
| | + | Followed by a shower, it helps you to feel wide awake (in the mornings/anytime). |

| | | |
|---|---|---|
| **Cycling:** | +/− | Low-injury (but only as long as other traffic users respect you). |
| | − | Some time is spent 'freewheeling' unless you choose your route carefully, so it may not have an aerobic effect for long enough. |
| | ? | Will you go out in all weathers? (Or, find an alternative aerobic exercise?) |

**Low-impact Aerobic exercise classes (dance; step):** are those where one foot always remains on the ground, unlike jumping, jogging, and running. It is a newer form of aerobics designed to minimise injury to joints. 'Low' does not indicate 'easier' or 'less effective', but should mean less risk of injury. So this form of aerobics is to be recommended, rather than the older type of aerobic jump/jog classes. Using a specially made step, to step up and down in a routine, is another new form of this sort of exercise. You need to purchase your 'step' to use.

Another variation of this type of exercise uses a 'Stretch Band' (rather like a giant-sized elastic band) to give resistance to your movements and make your body work harder, and your exercise more effective. (Videos also available.)

Classes vary very much in quality, so you need to choose carefully. Check for classes which have:
− A qualified and experienced teacher.
− A teacher who checks the correctness of your activities rather than

merely posing in front of a mirror preening and admiring her/himself.
- Not too many class members for proper supervision. If the instructor can't see you, you could be making mistakes and injuring yourself.
- A warm-up time, twenty minutes continuous aerobic work, a check on your pulse level and a cool-down set of exercise. If a section of 'stretching' exercises are included, too, so much the better.
- Music that's not too loud. Doctors are reporting increasing problems with hearing thought to be due to excessive zeal with the decibels.

**Low-Impact Aerobic Exercise videos:** These, too, vary in the quality of exercises, and are also subject to personal preferences for music and presentation. For example, I can't abide trendy Californians whooping and ow-ing their way through routines, yet other women enjoy it.

**Swimming:**
+ Minimal injury (as long as there's a life-guard!).
+ Good for litheness as well as its aerobic content.
? Only achieves aerobic effect if you swim *hard*.
? Is there a convenient pool?

**Aqua-aerobics:**
+ Minimal injury.
+ Great for those who fear water. You don't have to venture out of your depth.

**Jogging:**
- Risk of injury to legs and ankles. Wear suitable shoes, and run on grass or soft ground. Maybe unsafe for lone women.
- Traffic can be a hazard.

**Running:**
- Risk of injury if not properly supervised. Wear suitable shoes, run on grass or soft ground. Join a women's running club for advice and support.

**Rowing:**
+ Good if you live convenient to a club.
? Use a home or gym machine (but less possible to read and entertain yourself at the same time!).

**Skiing:**
+ But very few of us can fit this into our lifestyle, weekly!

**HOW OFTEN?** Three to four times per week. No less, for optimal effect. Heart fitness cannot improve with less. Even better, exercise up to six times per week.

You can combine from the above choices.

My favourite is the exercise bike and a good book. It tones and tightens the thighs and calf-muscles beautifully. Such bikes can be expensive, but are often advertised second-hand by people who make the mistake of asking themselves whether or not they'll bike today. (Unlike you, who will Just Do It.) Otherwise you could put an advertisement under a 'Miscellaneous Wanted' column of your local newspaper.

Check that the bike:
– is stable
– has some method of making the load heavier, as you become fitter
– has a reasonably comfortable seat (or get a cushion)
– doesn't have moving handlebars which you have to push, if you want to read a book. If you are willing to push the handlebars for 20–30 minutes, congratulations and carry on.

My other favourite form of exercise is the low-impact aerobic dance class. Despite there being many a winter's night after a hard day at work when I have a hate session about how impossible it is to move my poor dying body out of an armchair, I thoroughly enjoy them, and always return home rejuvenated and lively. I know that however tired I feel before I go, I shall feel a million per cent better afterwards.

## BECOMING LEAN: AEROBIC ACTIVITY PLAN

| Intensity of exercise: | Warm-up exercise | Aerobic exercise | Cool-down exercise | Relaxation |
| --- | --- | --- | --- | --- |
| Timing *Essential*: or up to: | 3–5 mins 10 mins | 20 mins 30 mins | 3–5 mins 10 mins | 3–5 mins 20 mins |
| Pulse rate: | Raising from normal resting rate | Within 'Target Zone' rate (see chart, page 214) | Dropping back towards normal resting | Lowered to normal, resting or even a little lower, at relaxation rate |

You are aiming, over a period of time, for a section of exercise that follows this format:
1 Warm-up:
   3–5 minutes essential (10 minutes, even better)
2 Aerobic section:
   20 minutes essential (30 minutes even better)
   Low-impact, high energy exercises
   Your pulse rate should be raised to your personal 'target zone'   (see pages 213-14)

3  Cool-down:
  3–5 minutes cool-down, lower-energy exercises
  Your pulse rate should drop back towards its 'normal' rate
4  Relaxation:
  3–5 minutes proper relaxation (up to 15–20 minutes would be lovely
if you have the time), preferably with some imagination-work that will
help your slimming, your motivation and your confidence. (You can buy
my cassette tape to help with this. See page 257.)

## BEGINNING AN AEROBIC EXERCISE PROGRAMME

For floor-based work, like an aerobics class, wear suitable footwear to
protect your feet and ankles from injury, and good socks. Don't do
aerobic dance exercise in just socks on a wood floor, because you may
slip. Consult a good sports shop; save your snack-money and present-
money if necessary, but do make it a priority to wear good trainer or
aerobic shoes.

Consult your doctor first if you:
– are very unfit
– are over two stones overweight
– have any medical condition
– are over 40 when you wish to begin.

Take this book to show him/her; tell him/her your plans, of exactly
what exercise you propose, for how long each time, and how often each
week. Ask for hishe/her comments; ask to have your blood pressure
checked, if he/she does not suggest it.

Ease into any exercise programme, following instructions about your
level of activity, and 'listen' to your body. If it's complaining, care for
it, and proceed more slowly. *Caution: excess exercise can be more
damaging than no exercise.*

## SUGGESTED BUILD-UP PROGRAMMES FOR AEROBIC EXERCISE

### 1  Exercise bike

WEEK 1

Warm-up: Easy 'load', 3 minutes.
Aerobic section: Increase 'load', 5 minutes.
Cool-down: Reduce load, 3 minutes.
Relaxation: 3 minutes.
TOTAL: 14 minutes, 3 times in week.

WEEKS 2–4

Increase the aerobic section to more than 5 minutes. Judge your own
fitness: try 10 minutes in week 2, then 15 minutes in weeks 3 and 4.
Increase to 20 minutes when you have checked your pulse rate (see page
214) and think that you can cope. Remember that you should be sweating,
and breathing heavily, but still able to hold a (puffy) conversation. If you
are too breathless to speak, or feel faint or sick, you are over-doing it.
Don't stop immediately, but slow down the activity gently to a stop.

## 2 Walking
WEEK 1
If you are very unfit, start with no more than 15 minutes. Increase your speed and time sensibly each week, according to your own fitness.
Warm-up: Walk at a fairly brisk pace, 5 minutes.
Aerobic section: Walk faster, with arms swinging, 5 minutes.
Cool down: Walk slower, as at the start, 5 minutes.
TOTAL: 15 minutes, 3 times in week.

For walking to produce an aerobic effect, most people need to walk at a speed of at least one mile in 20 minutes, aiming for one mile in 15 minutes. Fitter people need to 'speed walk' to 5–6 miles per hour, ie one mile in 10–12 minutes. Move that derriere and those arms!

Check off a mile in a car, or buy a pedometer from a sports shop. (You could tell your family that a pedometer is a more useful present for you than a box of chocolates.)
WEEKS 2–4
Increase the aerobic faster-walk section, to more than 5 minutes. Judge your own fitness; try 10 minutes in week 2, then 15 minutes in week 3 and 4. Increase to 20 minutes when you have checked your pulse rate and think that you can cope. Remember that you should be sweating, and breathing heavily, but still able to hold a (puffy) conversation. If you are too breathless to speak, or feel faint or sick, you are over-doing it. Don't stop immediately, but slow down the activity gently to a stop.

## 3 Swimming
Forget any worries about any excess weight, and if you can't swim, join a class, whatever your age. In Britain, many local authority pools now open early, to accommodate people before going to work.
Warm-up: Swim at a fairly brisk pace, 5 minutes
Aerobic section: Swim faster, with extra effort in both arms and legs, 5 minutes.
Cool down: Swim slower, as at the start, 5 minutes.
TOTAL: 15 minutes, 3 times in week.

For swimming to produce an aerobic effect, most people need to swim quite quickly. Check your pulse rate (see page 214) to discover whether you are getting valuable aerobic exercise.

Vary your stroke style to avoid boredom, and to increase your pulse rate: breast stroke is least work, the crawl is harder, and 'butterfly' is the most strenuous.
WEEKS 2–4
Increase the aerobic, faster section, to more than 5 minutes. Judge your own fitness; try 10 minutes on week 2; then 15 minutes weeks 3 and 4. Increase to 20 minutes when you have checked your pulse rate and think that you can cope. Remember that you should be sweating and breathing heavily, but still able, if you stopped, to hold a (puffy) conversation. If you are too breathless to speak, or feel faint or sick, you are over-doing it. Don't stop immediately, but slow down the activity gently to a stop.

**Aquarobics**
Some pools now offer these classes, which consist of exercises done in the water, often with one foot on the floor, usually not out of your depth. For it to be effective aerobic exercise, you need to be working fairly hard with leg and arm movements, and to be following the general timing guidelines as above. In London, Aquarobics Ltd will offer information on classes (Tel: 081 780 0870). Or you could construct your own programme by referring to the book *Aquarobics* by Glenda Baum (Arrow books).

**FINAL POINTS**
- Also, build activity into your day: eg use stairs not elevators, walk instead of driving or catching a bus.
- *Plan*: use the Planner which follows.
- Ease gently into any exercise programme.
- Persevere. The benefits of exercise take a while to show.
- Think Slim: exercise is a slimming friend!
- Repeat your Think Slim prompts while you are walking, swimming, cycling or treadmilling. Fit in the words rhythmically with your movements, and the thoughts will be fixed more firmly into your mind. Then the helpful prompts will be ready to emerge during the later crucial moments when you need inspiration.

**More experienced/fit exercisers**: should work-up, within the range of 60 per cent to 75 per cent as shown. As you become more fit, you can work higher up the range towards 85 per cent. Do *not* exercise harder or you may damage your heart.

Your exercise level should allow you to breathe heavily, and sweat, but still be able to talk. If you are not at all breathless, your exercise level is too low. If you are so breathless that you can't speak, or you feel sick or dizzy, you are overdoing it, so slow down immediately, and adjust your exercise so that your pulse rate stays within your target zone.

**PULSE RATE**
Your pulse rate 'target zone' is calculated by:
1 Subtract your age from 220. For example, a person 35 years old: 220–35=185
2 then calculate 60 per cent to 85 per cent of that figure. For example 185: 120–157.

To check your pulse rate, locate the beat at your wrist, with two fingers of the other hand. Count the number of beats, counting the first beat as 0, for 10 seconds; multiply this number by 6 to obtain the beats per minute.

Practise this often, so that you can locate and count it easily.

Alternatively, for convenience, purchase a pulse meter. These are made in wristwatch style, with a monitoring attachment for a finger, or ear. Available at good sport shops.

## IMPROVED FITNESS

The simple way of checking your improvement in cardio-vascular fitness is by noticing when your current level of exercise no longer raises your pulse as much as it did earlier.

If you want a more precise check, you can measure your progress by checking your pulse's 'recovery rate'. That is the rate at which your pulse drops back, after aerobic exercise. Cool down your exercise, and at the end of five minutes your pulse rate should have dropped back to below 120. The closer towards its resting, normal count, the fitter you appear to be.

Even more detail can be monitored: follow your cool-down exercises with a period of five minutes' proper relaxation, and check your pulse rate; greater fitness is indicated by the closeness of your pulse to its normal resting count. When you are even fitter, this may then be achieved in three minutes.

Your resting, normal pulse rate can be checked when you are sitting, resting; not immediately after exercise, eating, smoking or drinking alcohol.

A resting pulse rate for a man is usually 72 beats per minute; for a woman about 82. The fitter your cardio-vascular system, the slower this rate. A very fit male athlete may have a pulse rate in the 50s.

There is no need to become obsessed with pulse-taking, or worry that your pulse-rate isn't 'good enough'. Becoming slim-fit is not a competition, nor another goal to be desperately achieved like an exam result. Even the very act of taking your pulse can raise it slightly, because of your effort and the slight stress it may create. The idea of monitoring your pulse rate is to help you, not give you something else to be anxious about. So, regard it as a useful guide, and choose how involved you wish to be in monitoring your fitness improvement.

## MEASURING AEROBIC EXERCISE

Effective aerobic exercise should raise your heart rate to within 60 to 85 per cent of its maximum recommended figure (suitable for your age), as measured by your pulse rate.

Regularly working at that appropriate level can, as well as burn up calories, increase your cardio-vascular (heart and circulation) fitness and increase your metabolic rate. Working at a lower intensity will give little or no improvement. Working at a higher intensity – raising your pulse rate over the suggested range – can do permanent damage to your heart and must be avoided.

A chart follows to enable you to easily find the pulse rate range suitable for you, but please note:

**Beginners** should exercise hard enough for their pulse rate to be just about 60 per cent of the maximum heart-rate level, which is indicated on the chart, for their age range.

## AEROBIC TRAINING EFFECT: TARGET PULSE COUNT CHART

| AGE | BEGINNERS | | EXPERIENCED | | | |
|---|---|---|---|---|---|---|
| | 60% OF MAXIMUM PULSE RATE | | 75% | to | | 85% |
| | 10 sec count | 1 min | 10 sec count | 1 min | 10 sec count | 1 min |
| 16–20 | 20 | 120 | 25 | 150 | 28 | 170 |
| 21–25 | 19 | 117 | 24 | 146 | 27 | 166 |
| 26–30 | 19 | 114 | 24 | 143 | 27 | 161 |
| 31–35 | 18 | 111 | 23 | 139 | 26 | 157 |
| 36–40 | 18 | 108 | 23 | 135 | 25 | 153 |
| 41–45 | 17 | 105 | 22 | 131 | 25 | 149 |
| 46–50 | 17 | 102 | 21 | 128 | 24 | 144 |
| 51–55 | 17 | 99 | 21 | 124 | 23 | 140 |
| 56–60 | 16 | 96 | 20 | 120 | 22 | 136 |
| 61–65 | 15 | 93 | 19 | 116 | 21 | 131 |
| 66–70 | 15 | 90 | 18 | 112 | 21 | 127 |
| 71–75 | 14 | 87 | 17 | 108 | 20 | 123 |
| 76–80 | 14 | 84 | 17 | 105 | 19 | 119 |
| 81–90 | 13 | 78 | 16 | 97 | 18 | 110 |

## 2 BECOMING LITHE

Being lithe is about being supple, able to bend, twist and turn easily without spraining or injuring our bodies as we go about our everyday lives. Whether pegging out the washing; hauling up the baby or a bed-resting convalescent aunt; clambering into a sports car, onto a horse or up a ladder to Do-It-Yourself; whether throwing the ball for the dog, playing cricket with the kids, or venturing into the world of the Karma Sutra with the lover in your life, being lithe increases the quality of our lives.

Getting older can mean joints getting stiffer, creakier and more susceptible to strains and backaches. If we don't want to lose our suppleness, we must use it. The good news is that in a tested experiment, people of over 40 improved their suppleness levels as much as did the twenty-somethings, given gentle practice. Dancers who are old by the count of their birthdays demonstrate their 'youthful' suppleness. Suppleness is not the prerogative of the young (indeed some young folk are noticeably un-supple), but it is the characteristic of those who work for it. (Remember the Think Slim: 'everything in life has to be paid for'.)

Becoming lithe doesn't have to take a lot of time, but it takes (as does every achievement) thought, planning and action. To become lithe, it's helpful to start by finding out how you are now.

## BECOMING LITHE: ASSESS YOURSELF

If you take time out to assess yourself just before you begin this exercise programme, you will have the pleasure of noting the improvement of your body's suppleness. Whatever your age or level of unfitness, you can improve suppleness. So, try these self-assessments, and fill in the charts so that you can compare them at one-month intervals. Don't fall into the Negative Wizard trap of berating yourself if you can't do these exercises very well at present. This is not a test for you to pass, it's merely a start-line indicator so that, later, you can be delighted with your improvement.

Before you start, warm up with three to five minutes of gentle-ish aerobic exercise (on your exercise bike, dancing, or feet tapping and arms swinging) to warm up your muscles. Don't do these assessments if your body is cold. Wear comfortable and warm-enough clothing which covers your legs if the room temperature is less than 70°F/21°C.

## 1 Side Bends

Stand, feet together, arms at your sides. Without bending either forwards or leaning back, reach down the side of your leg with your hand.

| Check | Answer | Date | Review Dates |
|---|---|---|---|
| With your right hand on your right side | | | |
|   Can you reach your knee? | .................... | ............. | ............. |
|   Notice how far down you can reach | .................... | ............. | ............. |
| With your left hand on your left side: | | | |
|   Can you reach your knee? | .................... | ............. | ............. |
|   Notice how far down you can reach | .................... | ............. | ............. |

## 2 Sit-stretch

Sit with legs together in front of you. Flex back your feet and toes towards your face. Don't jerk or strain, but reach forward with your hands to touch, or pass, your toes.

| | | | |
|---|---|---|---|
| Can you touch your toes? (If not, note to where you can reach.) | .................... | ............. | ............. |
| Can you reach past your toes: with your knuckles? | .................... | ............. | ............. |

with the whole length of your
fingers?                                    ......................    ..............    ..............
with half way down your palm?    ......................    ..............    ..............
with the whole of your palm?     ......................    ..............    ..............

## 3  Calf Stretch

Sit in the same position, but with your feet flexed against a wall. Keeping your heels still, can you flex back your toes so that there is a space about 2 inches/5 cm from the wall?

Can you flex back the toes to leave
any space between the wall and
your toes?                                  ......................    ..............    ..............
Can you leave a space of about 2
inches/5 cm?                                ......................    ..............    ..............

## 4  Thigh Stretch

Lie down on your stomach. Bend your knees and push your heel towards your buttock. Gently, with the same-side hand, push your heel to touch your buttock.

Can you push your right heel to
touch your buttock? (If not, how
far off, approximately, are you?
Check in a mirror, or ask a friend.)     ......................    ..............    ..............

Can you push your left heel to your
buttock? If so, *without straining* try
this:
    Can you lift your right foot up a
    little with your right hand so that
    your knee comes off the floor
    about a couple of inches?              ......................    ..............    ..............
    Can you lift your left foot up a
    little with your left hand so that
    your knee comes off the floor
    a couple of inches?                    ......................    ..............    ..............

## 5  Shoulder Touch

Take your right arm straight up by your ear, fold the elbow so the right hand slides down your back. Keep your left arm down by your left side, and fold it up your back. Keep your left arm down by your left side, and fold it up your back at the elbow. *Without* undue strain:

Can you meet/touch the fingers
together?                                   ......................    ..............    ..............

Repeat with opposite arms; that is, your left arm up by your ear, and your right hand folded up your back.
Can you meet/touch the fingers together? (If not, you need a friend to tell you

how far away you are; check each side as it is quite usual to have one side more supple than the other. If you are a long way off, you can hold a scarf in your top hand and grasp that with the lower hand.)

## BECOMING LITHE: ESSENTIAL EXERCISES:

Wear warm-enough clothing; legs covered (unless it is hot weather or a very warm room); socks and suitable trainer shoes or barefoot if it's warm enough; and work in a reasonable room-temperature.

Warm-Up: always warm-up the body first, to prevent strain or injury. Do either, three to five minutes on an exercise bike, at a speed and load that makes you breathe heavily and begin to sweat. Or, five minutes 'rag doll' dancing to up-beat music: let your body loose and move like a rag doll, shaking and swinging arms and legs (not jogging) so that you breathe heavily and begin to sweat. The longer the warm-up, the better. Ten minutes is better than five.

*Only then*, begin the following exercises. In the 'Standing' posture, do not arch your back. Stand straight, but don't over-correct like a sergeant major.

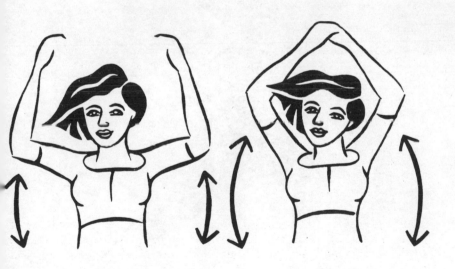

## 1 Shoulders: standing position

Shrug your shoulders up and down: 8 times
Shrug your shoulders *gently* backwards: 4 times
Shrug your shoulders *gently* forwards: 4 times
Gently and loosely, swing both arms up from your sides, firstly, as high as shown, 4 times; then, into a full circle: 4 times.

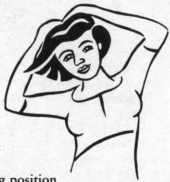

## 2  Side Body Stretch: standing position

Stand with feet comfortably apart, hands held up by your head. Without leaning forward or back, bend over to the left, and hold the stretch that you feel on the opposite side, for three seconds; release back to standing position. Do this three to five times on each side.

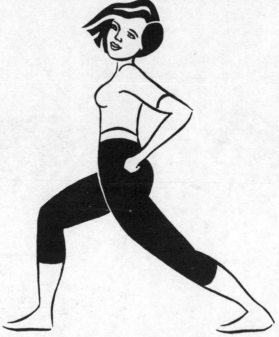

## 3  Calf Stretch: standing position

Stand with hands on hips. Place one foot forward of the other (feet straight, not turned out), slightly bending the front knee, and the back leg straight (but not locked tight) with your rear foot flat on the floor. You feel the stretch in your calf; hold for three seconds. Change legs; and repeat, three to five times with each leg.

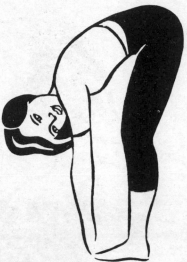

## 4 Roll Down: standing position

Stand, feet comfortably apart, knees comfortably straight but not locked tight. Stretch both arms high up above your head, stretching up the ribs, too. Slowly and gently roll your arms and body down, fingers towards the floor, *without jerking or bouncing*. Try to touch the floor. Hold for three seconds. Roll up gently. Repeat three to five times.

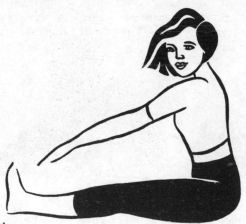

## 5 Sit-Stretch: sitting position

Sit with legs together, forward in front of you. Flex back your feet, toes towards your face. Don't jerk or strain, but reach forward with your hands to touch, or pass, your toes.

This is the same exercise as in the self-assessment. Check how much further you can comfortably stretch, over time. The aim is to improve at your body's own pace, not to compete with others or push yourself.

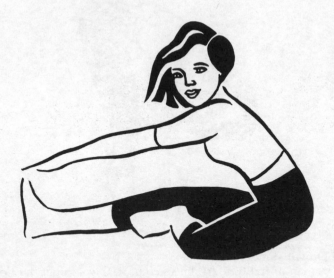

## 6  Hamstring Stretch: sitting position

Sit with legs wide apart. Bend your right leg so that your foot is touching the other knee. Leave your other leg straight out, but don't lock the knee tight. Gently curl your upper body, and lean forward over the straight leg, to touch your foot, or as near as you can get. Hold the stretch for three seconds. Repeat three to five times. Change legs and repeat on the other side.

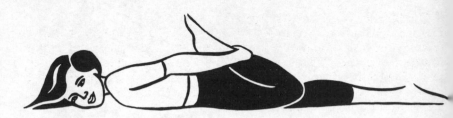

## 7  Thigh Stretch: lying on stomach position

Lie on your stomach. Bend your right knee, and push your heel towards your buttock. Gently, with the same side hand, push your heel to touch your buttock. You should feel the stretch along the front of the thigh of your bent leg. Hold for three seconds. Change legs, and repeat. Repeat three to five times on each leg.

This is the same exercise as in the self-assessment. Check how much further you can comfortably push your heel, and stretch, over time.

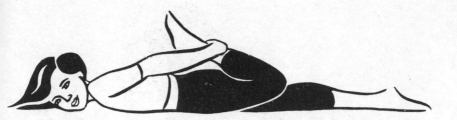

If this exercise is, or becomes, easy for you, move on to the next level. Without straining, gently lift your left foot with your left hand so that your knee comes off the floor about a couple of inches/5 cm. Don't move on to this level until you feel your body is really ready to do so.

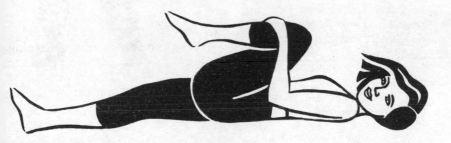

**8 Hip Stretch: lying on back position**
Lie on your back with your legs out straight. Bring your right leg up towards your chest. Put your hands around this knee, and gently pull it towards your chest. (Don't jerk or force or cause pain.) Hold for ten seconds, breathing slowly. Try to pull the knee a little closer. Hold the closer position for 10 seconds, breathing slowly. Repeat with the other leg. Repeat three to five times on each.

## 3 BECOMING MAGNIFICENT
Perhaps this is rather an over-the-top description. But let's abandon our reserve, and allow ourselves to become and feel at least a bit magnificent.

The lion and lioness have muscles toned to magnificence by their jungle lifestyle, but we 'civilised society' folk have to tone and tighten our muscles by exercises designed for the purpose.

Most women seem to want to tone their waist, tum and thighs, and these are the areas on which this programme concentrates.

# BECOMING MAGNIFICENT: ESSENTIAL TONE AND TIGHTEN EXERCISES

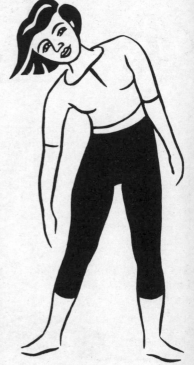

### 1 Waist Toner: standing position
Stand with feet comfortably apart, slightly turned out, arms at your sides. Without bending either forwards or backwards, reach down the side of your leg with your left hand, 20 times. Repeat on the other side with your right hand. You are aiming to reach your knee, and then beyond. Don't jerk down to reach further; allow yourself to improve sensibly, over time, with practice.

Increase from 20 to 40 times for more improvement.

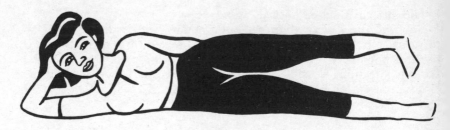

### 2 Thigh Toner: lying-on-side position
Lie on your side, as in a straight line, supporting your upper body on your bent elbow. Using the top leg, flex the foot, pointing your toes towards your face; and move the leg up and down (about 10 inches) without resting back on the other foot. Keep the leg straight, without bending the knee. Move the leg up and down 20 to 30 times, but start with as few as eight times if this exercise is new to you.

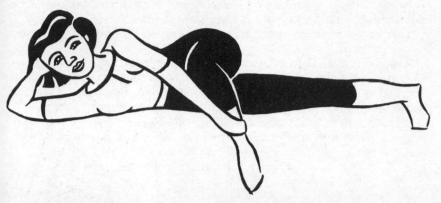

Then put the top leg over in front of the other, foot forward, holding the foot with your hand if you need to (see picture). Flex the foot of the underneath leg, and raise the leg as high as possible, without bending the knee, up and down but without touching the floor. Move the leg up and down 20 to 25 times, but start with as few as eight times if this exercise is new to you.

Lie on your other side, and repeat.

### 3 Tummy-Crunch Tightener: lying-on-back position

Lie on your back. Bend your knees, putting your feet flat on the floor, about the width of your hips apart. Press the middle of your back into the floor. Do not arch your back. Check whether you can get your hands under your middle back; you shouldn't be able to. If you can, you are still arching your back, and need to flatten it out.

Choose your arm/hand position:

Beginners: the easiest position for your hands is arms forward, hands pointing towards your knees.

Second level: arms crossed over your chest.

Hardest: arms bent up, hands by your ears. Do *not* clasp your hands behind your head, or pull your neck as you can injure yourself this way.

You must not jerk, bounce or go at speed, with this exercise. Macho-types in a gym often demonstrate these crunches with great speed but with no thought for the state of their spines. The aim is not to massage your ego, but to tighten your stomach muscles, safely.

So, aim to 'sit up' only so far as taking your shoulder blades off the ground. Remember these features:

– Press your middle back into the floor – don't arch it.

– Keep your chin in as 'normal' a position as possible. Don't tuck it into your chest.

– Don't pull your neck round and forward. Keep it as normal as possible, or you will have a strained neck and a still-flabby tum.

– Keep your eyes on the ceiling to help to keep your chin and neck uncurled.

– Never do tummy-crunch type exercises with legs straight out. You may damage your back. *Always* have knees bent.
– Tighten your tummy muscles just before you lift yourself into your tummy-crunch.

With knees bent, arms in chosen position and tum tight, lift your upper body only up as far as your shoulder blades off the floor; then lower it again. Don't hook your feet under something to help you; the 'something' will be doing the work instead of your tummy muscles.

If you can hardly move yourself upwards, don't worry – practise five at a time, frequently (preferably twice every day). You *can* improve with practice. Aim to do eight, then increase towards 30; that is, three sets of ten: 10 crunches, 10 seconds rest; 10 crunches, 10 seconds rest; 10 crunches, 10 seconds rest.

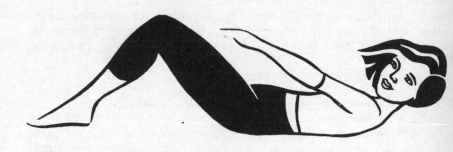

These 30 will take you less than three minutes each day, and you will be delighted with the result. (No, not by next Saturday!) Persevere for three months, along with your Slimfit eating programme, and you can enjoy a magnificent improvement in the trimness of your stomach. It is the only exercise that I heartily recommend to be done every day (or six out of seven days). It's the most rewarding way of spending three minutes every day (well, almost – certainly for improving your figure). Build the tummy-crunches into your morning routine, (after your exercise bike and shower?). They are no more difficult to include than cleaning your teeth.

## AN EFFORTLESS WAY TO TONE UP?
If you are still tempted to think that there is *any* effortless way to become slim and fit, think again.

Even toning tables are not totally passive. For results, you are usually expected to use your own muscles as resistance to the table movement. Toning tables do not generally claim to get you slimmer or make you lose weight. Many salons offer a diet sheet (excuse my cynical smile), for following a diet sheet may be more responsible for many of the extravagant claims of 'inches lost' than reclining on the table. Also, measuring accurately around tum, hips, thighs and calves is notoriously difficult; how can you be absolutely sure the tape is in exactly the same place next time? Test this at home, and see what variations you can get!

Toning tables can, at best, do no more than 'tone' your muscles. It's a very expensive way to tone up, and for most people, probably not worth it. On the other hand, if you've got the money to spare, you don't expect miracles, and you enjoy it – go ahead. Tessa went for a course to help her to 'keep in the mood for slimming'; it helped her motivation, and helped her to break her evening television-and-sweets routine. It may be relaxing, and meeting other women who are interested in being fitter and slimmer can be pleasant, too. (As long as you don't sympathise pathetically with each other about how hard it all is . . .) It's your money; you decide whether, on balance, it's worth it for you.


## LEAN, LITHE AND MAGNIFICENT: PUTTING YOUR TOTAL BODYPOWER PROGRAMME TOGETHER

Action cannot begin without thought. As this programme recognises you as an individual with individual needs and wants, the final putting-it-all-together plan must be thought out by you. However, help is at hand: a recap on the three aspects of the BodyPower Programme:

A combination of:

| 1<br>LOW-IMPACT AEROBIC EXERCISE | 2<br>LITHENESS EXERCISES | 3<br>TONE AND TIGHTEN EXERCISES |
|---|---|---|
| Suggested per week:<br>3–4 times | 2–3 times | 2–3 times |
| Up to:<br>6 times | 4 times | 6 times |
| Choose from the aerobic list: eg bike, swim, walk, work-out class or video | 8 litheness exercises | Tummy Crunches, thigh, and waist exercise |

Some of the exercises perform more than one function. For example, an exercise bike will tone thighs and calves as well as be aerobic; aerobic swimming and walking can also help litheness; a well-balanced aerobic dance session can promote suppleness as well as tone and tighten.

**Litheness**: You don't have to do all the eight exercises every time, if you don't wish to. Choose the ones to improve your least supple areas.

**Tone and tighten**: The Tummy Crunch exercises are recommended six times per week, every day except for one rest day. They are very quick to do, yet very effective; less than three minutes for 30. A good return on your investment of time.

The thigh exercises would not be needed at all if you use an exercise bike at least 3 times per week.

Construct your weekly programme, selecting from each of the three exercise groups. Use the Planner which follows.

## EXERCISE PLANNER

If you think you 'might' do 'some' exercise, 'some' day – some chance! If you *think*, and *plan*, it's much more likely that you will *do*. This Planner is designed to be used by you to plan your exercise for the week. Copy it out for a few weeks until your exercise routine *becomes* routine.

Firstly, below, there is a filled-in example to show you the idea.

This week I shall exercise as follows:

|  | AEROBIC |  | LITHENESS STRETCH | TONE & TIGHTEN |
|---|---|---|---|---|
| Type of Exercise | exercise bike | aerobic class | all 8 exercises | tummy-crunches |
| How much | 20 min |  |  | 10 |
| Days | Mon, Wed, Fri | Thurs | Tues | every day |
| Time | am before work | 8 pm | am before work | am before work after shower |

NB: Some exercise, such as swimming, can be both aerobic and for litheness. Put it in its 'main' column; this is not a 'purist' chart. It is a Planner to help you.

This week I shall exercise as follows:

| | Aerobic | Litheness Stretch | Tone & Tighten |
|---|---|---|---|
| Type of Exercise | | | |
| How much | | | |
| Days | | | |
| Time | | | |

# THINK SLIM QUIZZES

## PROMPTS QUIZ

Throughout this book, Think Slim phrases have been presented. It is important that such Think Slim becomes part of your everyday thinking. Check yourself with this 'complete the gaps' quiz to see how many of these Think Slim phrases you have remembered. The completed list can be found on page 266. This list can also be used for you to make your personal Think Slim Prompt Cards. (Each dash equals one letter.)

### FUNDAMENTAL THINK SLIM

1 The key to being slim is: _ _ _ _ _ _ _ _ _.
2 I _ _ _ _ _ therefore I am . . . slim-fit.
3 Life – This is Not A D_ _ _ _ R_ _ _ _ _ _ _ _. Live now, there is no 'later'.
4 Life in the Fat Lane is life in s_ _ _ m_ _ _ _ _.
5 Slim-fit living is more en_ _ _ _ _ _ _ living.
6 Life isn't _ _ _ _.
7 Nobody promised me that life would be _ _ _ _.
8 Choosing to do one thing often means choosing _ _ _ to do another.
9 Everything in life is _ _ _ _ _ _ said than done.

### ON EATING

1 'A _ _ _ _ _ _ of What You Fancy does You Good!' (A _ _ _ _ _ _ only: a _ _ _ makes you Fat!)
2 Think before you eat a TH _ _ _.
3 If the _ _ _ _'_ not fabulous, don't _ _ _ _ _ the calories on it!
4 Those who _ _ _ _ - _ _ _ _ _ _ _ _ – bulge!
5 You'll get more p_ _ _ _ _ _ _ out of being slim than you ever got from _ _ _ _ - _ _ _ _ _ _.
6 It's just as f_ _ _ _ _ _ _ _ if you eat it in s_ _ _ _ _.
7 Linger l_ _ _ _ _ with your food. Get more p_ _ _ _ _ _ _ out of l_ _ _ calories.

8 Food can't solve p_ _ _ _ _ _. Only I can do that.

9 More f_ _ _ can only make me more f_ _.

10 I give up to _ _ _.

## ON SLIMMING

1 We are overweight because we _ _ _ _ - _ _ _!

2 Make ef_ _ _ _ _ – not ex_ _ _ _ _.

3 It's not sl_ _ _ _ _ _ _ that's miserable – it's being _ _ _!

4 Deprived. Who's m_ _ _ deprived? (The slim person who deprives herself only of over-eating – *or* the fat one who eats anything and everything and deprives herself of the pleasures of being slim?)

5 Successful slimmers m_ _ _ it happen; disastrous dieters l_ _ it happen.

## ON FAILURE

1 You won't know where you're going, if you're always l_ _ _ _ _ _ back!

2 You haven't failed until you s_ _ _ tr_ _ _ _!

## ON EATING OUT

1 I've paid for it, I've got to eat it. No! I've paid for it so I can d_ wh_ _ I l_ _ _ w_ _ _ it – and that includes l_ _ _ _ _ _ it!

Answers on page 266.

# QUIZ: HOW MUCH HAVE YOU LEARNED SO FAR?

This is not a test! It is simply for you to check out how much you have learned so far, to help you be more effective in your slimming.

Some of the following Think Slim sentences have words missing. Check how much you have learned so far, by trying to remember the words that are missing. There are also questions. Check your knowledge by thinking of the answers.

If you have a 'Think Slimming' friend you could work these out together and then discuss the topics.

(Each dash equals one letter.)

1 We are overweight because we _ _ _ _ - _ _ _.

2 We should keep on weighing our _ _ _ _, NOT _ _ _ _ _ _ _ _ _.

3 It's good to make resolutions and set targets, but these should be _ _ _ _ _ _ _ _ _.

4 Lil is plagued by a Negative Wizard in herself; she used to think: 'That li'l bit won't _ _ _ _!'
Was she right?

  5 An extra _ _ calories a day could amount to over 4 stones/25 kilos of weight gain in 10 years.
6 How many calories in one peanut?
  In one grape?
  Which product has the least amount of calories: butter, margarine, polyunsaturated spread (such as Flora)? About how many calories are in 1 oz/28 g?
7 Motivation is essential for slimming action. Motivation spurs us into action, and begins from our thinking. Two important motivators are: Think W_ _, and Think P_ _ _ _ _ _.
8 Two words/phrases, beginning with P, are MOST important for slimmers; we need to educate ourselves to have both of these. What are they? (Per_ _ _ _ _ _ _ _ and Pos_ _ _ _ _ At_ _ _ _ _ _).
  9 Why is it a good idea for slimmers to take a vitamin and mineral tablet each day? Are you taking yours?!
10 DO'S AND DON'TS!
  Don't b_ _ _ yourself with cottage cheese and carrots all week!
  Don't make yourself mis_ _ _ _ _ _ over a small weight loss.
  Do think that you are 'on the r_ _ _ _ tr_ _ _!'
  Any (sensible) weight loss is a _ _ _ _ loss.
  Do drink enough liquids (low-calorie). How many mugs each day?
  Do make your eating HIGH-F_ _ _ _! Why?
  And by eating which foods?
11 Have you felt hungry this week?
  How did you know that you were hungry?
  What did you do about it?


Answers on page 267.

# PART II
# BECOMING SLIM-FIT

# THE
# WAS–IS STORIES:
## Some examples of
## successful Think Slimmers

*IRENE*
Age: 40
Height: 5 feet 1 inch/1.55 metres
Was: 10 stones 7 pounds/66.7 kilos
Is: 8 stones 12 pounds/56.2 kilos
Weight Lost: 1 stone 8 pounds/10 kilos

**Lifestyle:** Irene lives in a village with her husband and two teenage sons. She works full-time as a teacher of adults who have learning difficulties, in a top-security mental hospital.

'Dolloping the double cream into exotic dishes, just as my beautiful cookbooks advised, started my weight problem, soon after I was married,' explains Irene. 'At first it was only 1 stone/6 kilos, but three pregnancies later, my just-married 9 stone slimness had ballooned to 11 stones (57 kilos to 70 kilos), and I was very unhappy about it.

'Over the next ten years, my weight see-sawed up and down, as I used one diet after another – all ruined by going back, in between, to my double-cream recipes and old eating habits.

'Like many women, I suffered from the "pear-shape" figure – slim from the waist upwards. I thought I was a "permanent pear".

'Then I joined Eve's group and changed my eating and thinking habits; I bought new cookbooks with delicious, low-fat recipes; I go to her exercise class and work out at home too; I cycle.'

Irene refused to allow a major operation and its forced inactivity to spoil her slimming. She had a little notice which read:

> *VISITORS*
> PLEASE **DO NOT** FEED UP THE PATIENT.
> NO CHOCOLATES OR GRAPES BY REQUEST.

'I wanted to be "8 stone-something",' she declares, 'and now I am!' (under 58 kilos). One and a half stones (10 kilos) may not seem like a lot of weight to have lost, yet the difference in Irene's figure is amazing; not a hint of pear-shape about her svelte hips, thighs and tum. A new curly hairstyle, plus trendy specs in psychedelic frames, completes her new look and earns her clutches of compliments.

Irene declares: 'I have no thoughts of going back to the fat old ways of eating or cooking, or thinking. I enjoy my life so much more. I love wearing fashionable clothes – and how great I felt one day when my teenage son shouted in surprise, seeing me in my new slinky black leggings: "Hey, Mum, you look just as good as Tina Turner!"'

### IRENE'S PERSONAL TIPS FOR YOU
**Think Slim:** 'Everything in life has to be paid for'.

Irene explains: 'This reminds me that nothing in life is achieved without effort, including being slim and fit. The benefits of being slim and fit are so good that if "effort" is the price, I'm prepared to pay.'
**Practical Tip:** 'If you have over-indulged, wear something quite tight, just to remind you that you have to make up for the over-indulgence! Because if you slip on something a little more comfortable, there's a danger you'll kid yourself that your weight is still OK, and you won't make the special effort needed to reduce it.'

## JULIE
Age: 21
Height: 5 feet 4 inches/1.63 metres
Was: 11½ stones/73 kilos
Is: 8 stones 13 pounds/56.7 kilos
Weight Lost: 2 stones 8 pounds/16 kilos

**Lifestyle:** Julie lives at home with her parents, and is engaged to be married soon. She works full time as a hairdresser, and in her spare time enjoys competition ballroom dancing.

'By the time I was in the third year at secondary school I was overweight,' remembers Julie. 'I didn't like it but I never really tried to do anything about it. I'd seen enough of my Mum with her diets! The food was always so horrible. She had one diet where she had to eat a cupful of beetroot each day – ugh!

'I thought if that's dieting, it's not for me! Then I tried Eve's slimming group and found a much better way to lose weight. I learned to get slim eating "normal" sorts of meals and to include my favourite foods in moderation. To succeed I also had to change how I think, especially about eating on impulse.'

Julie's ballroom dancing hobby includes Latin American Sequence style. She says: 'I used to come off the floor after only one dance, gasping for breath! Now I've plenty of energy to keep going, and I know I present myself better now I'm slim. We win more awards these days, too!'

Soon it will be one of the most important days of Julie's life: her wedding day. When she glides down that aisle, she can be confident that she will look beautiful in her romantic fashionable dress with its tiny waist and its billowing skirt. Julie comments: 'I'm so glad that I lost my weight long before my wedding. It's lovely to be getting married in a size 10 dress. Those wedding photos will last forever, and I'm so pleased I shan't look like a lump of lard in white!'

Mum gave up those crazy diets, and lost almost 2 stones/12½ kilos at my slimming group, along with Julie, so she is thrilled that she will be an elegant slim 'mother of the bride'. The bridegroom? He thinks Julie's slim-fitness is just great.

## JULIE'S PERSONAL TIPS FOR YOU

**Think Slim:** 'I always keep this little rhyme in my mind when I think about eating (especially when I wander, in boredom, to the fridge): 'Do I really want it? Not I don't. Shall I eat it? No I won't!'

**Practical Tip:** 'I always totalled up the calories I had eaten, at the end of the day, and if I had any left from my 1000 allowance, I spent them on something for a light supper.' With the Think Slim Eating Programme you don't have to count calories, but if you think it might help you, as it did Julie, you can do so.

# MARY
Age: 38
Height: 5 feet 3 inches/1.60 metres
Was: 13 stones 4 pounds/84.4 kilos
Is: 10 stones 4 pounds/65 kilos
Weight Lost: 3 stones/19 kilos (and still slimming)

**Lifestyle:** Mary lives with her husband in a very large village, and works full-time in a city in a training agency.

'I was always what they call a "bonny" child,' laughs Mary, 'but as a teenager, that weight just rolled off and I was a reasonably slim 9½ stones/60 kilos when I got married at 23 years old.

'But then,' she continues, 'I thought that being a good wife meant I ought to feed hubby up, puddings and all. Of course, I fed myself up, too. My weight crept up gradually and I never kept a check on it – just bought larger clothes! Then came the day that I shopped for a black velvet skirt, and found that I needed a size 20. That did it. I came out of the shop with no skirt, but determined to lose weight.'

So, Mary joined one of my slimming groups, and has just a few more pounds to lose to reach her chosen target weight. She tells how. 'I've changed how I think and live. I used to crave chocolate and eat it all at once; now I know I can have some if I want, and I can eat a bit and leave it. I used to sit, and sit and sit, and eat and eat and eat. But now I've more energy and do more things. I used to be breathless and worn out after walking the dog, yet now I'm ready to get on with something else. I enjoy lots of compliments, especially from my husband, and more cuddles from him too . . .'

Hubby doesn't mind the lack of puds, for he also has lost weight (1 stone/6 kilos), and, anyway, they do enjoy puds as *occasional* treats on Mary's 'Think Slim' principles.

Oh, and that black velvet skirt? Slim-fit Mary now wears an elegant straight style in a size 14, and will soon need it to be altered to a size 12. How does it feel?

'Marvellous!' enthuses Mary. 'I'll never go back to how I used to live.'

## MARY'S PERSONAL TIPS FOR YOU

**Think Slim:** 'Whenever you are tempted to eat by thinking "That Li'l Bit Won't Hurt" think again, and don't eat.'

Mary says: 'I learned to think about what I ate between meals, and also about my nibbling when packing up lunch sandwiches for hubby and myself.' She removed this fattening habit by Thinking Slim every time she was tempted to nibble; she also reminds herself of a little saying brought to our group by another slimmer: 'Little Pickers wear Big Knickers'. Mary is no longer a 'Little Picker'. Nor does she wear . . .

**Practical Tip:** 'Never fry your food. Eat more fruit and vegetables to satisfy your appetite. Do have favourite treats – but *occasionally.*'

## JENNY

Age: 50-something
Height: 5 feet 4 inches/1.63 metres
Was: 14 stones 7 pounds/92 kilos
Is: 9 stones 7 pounds/60 kilos
Weight Lost: 5 stones/32 kilos

**Lifestyle:** Jenny lives with her husband, whom she married over thirty years ago, and her two grown-up sons. A third son lives independently. She never worked all her married life until she lost her excess weight and then she got a part-time job as a school lunch-time supervisor; now she works as a 'Lollipop lady', helping school-children to cross busy roads.

'I don't think I'll ever be able to do that!' commented Jenny ruefully, the very first time she saw the other ladies performing their aerobic dance exercises at one of my slimming groups. But Jenny soon learned to banish such negative thoughts, and to Think Slim instead. Nowadays, weighing less by five stones/32 kilos, she still comes to my 'work-out' class, and goes dancing three other evenings.

'I took your advice – to get out and Do Something instead of staying in and eating,' she comments, 'and I really enjoy life now.' I've more confidence than I ever dreamed I could have. I've altered my whole outlook on life. I'm a really different person.'

Jenny had always been fat, ever since she was a child. All her adult life she had tried dieting, but always bounced back to her old bad eating habits and high weight. The only time she lost weight successfully was when her doctor gave her amphetamine slimming pills (no longer prescribed) so she was slim on her wedding day. But slimming drugs do not teach you to stay slim, and she was soon fat again. Joining the Think Slim group changed all that.

'I dithered about starting,' she admits. 'My son took me, and left me outside, so I plucked up courage to come in. The ideas were so *encouraging*, I found I could succeed.'

She has kept that slim and fit figure for over three years, and loves her different, better lifestyle. Jenny vows: 'I'll never go back to being fat.'

### JENNY'S PERSONAL TIPS FOR YOU

**Think Slim:** 'It isn't slimming that's miserable – it's being fat! I avoided feeling sorry for myself when I needed to say no to some foods by remembering that I was, at last, doing something to solve my fat problem.'

**Practical Tip:** 'Serve your meals on a smaller plate than you have usually used. Your portions look larger and are more satisfying to your eye and your brain.'

With a husband and two sons who are all hefty eaters, this has been a big help to Jenny, and even if you don't share your table with men who can eat more than you, you could still find that Jenny's tip helps you.

## PAT

Age: 56
Height: 5 feet 4 inches/1.63 metres
Was: 9 stones 10 pounds/61.7 kilos
Is: 7 stones 10 pounds/50 kilos
Weight Lost: 2 stones/11.7 kilos

**Lifestyle:** Pat lives with her husband on the outskirts of a market town, and is a working partner with him in their own business, a residential home for elderly people. She has one son who is married and who, just over a year ago, made her a grandmother to Luke.

'I used to be complimented that I didn't look my age, but when you get overweight you *do* look your age. And feel it,' begins Pat. 'I always used to be trim without much effort, all my life, at about 8½ stones/54 kilos,' she explains, 'but then we sold our business (another residential home), and I stayed at home and the weight just went on. In the business, I had been running up and down stairs and lifting those who weren't able . . .

using many extra calories that being at home didn't do. I tried cutting down on my food, and even went on those Very Low Calorie Liquid Diets. One didn't suit me at all, and I was often sick; with another I lost a very little weight, but it returned very quickly.

'I despaired. I gave away some lovely pairs of trousers which were just too small. I thought, it's no use, I'll never get in those again!

'With Eve's slimming group I learned to think before I ate, and consider what calories I was about to put in my mouth; yet I could still include my favourite small ice cream bar – 70 calories – most evenings.'

Pat has always loved dressing smartly, and now looks and feels better than ever; she's a very elegant grandmother.

'I also like to wear tiny bikini briefs, without any flabby overhang,' she adds.

Pat and Ron have just started another residential home, for they didn't enjoy retirement, and she has plenty of slim-fit energy to offer. She doesn't regret giving away those trousers, for now they'd be too big for her toned-up figure. And she felt good when, recently, her son called to say: 'Mum, help me get some weight off – please tell me what to do!'

## PAT'S PERSONAL TIPS FOR YOU
**Think Slim:** 'Is it worth its Calories?'

Pat explains: 'When I am about to eat something, I always think to myself whether the food is worth its calories. Crisps used to be my weakness but now I think to myself that they are *not* worth what they are going to do to my figure!'

**Practical Tip:** 'Change the balance of your meals; less meat, more vegetables. I combine interesting veg in the microwave, such as tomatoes, courgettes, broccoli and onions. A tasty and low-fat filler.

## DONNA
Age: 24
Height: 5 feet 3 inches/1.60 metres
Was: 9 stones 5 pounds/59.42 kilos
Is: 8 stones 2½ pounds/51.94 kilos
Weight Lost: 1 stone 2½ pounds/7.48 kilos

**Lifestyle:** Donna qualified as a hairdresser but nowadays she stays at home caring for her step-daughter, aged five, and her baby who is a year old. She and her family, including husband Les, live in a large village. Donna is also registered as a Child Minder but currently is not 'minding'.

'Now I'm *back to normal*!' whooped Donna in delight, as the weighing scales confirmed she had reached her chosen target weight. Like many women, Donna had found that, after baby Katie was born, her weight did not naturally return to 'normal'.

'I felt fat,' she confides, 'and miserable about it. Also, I found myself needing to ask Les if he still loved me, whereas when I was slim I felt quite confident about it. Now he often tells me how wonderful I look. I know I look good . . . and I feel good about it. I had been a chubby child and I was teased about it at school. My parents used to urge me to eat, eat, eat, because they didn't like waste, and I obeyed them.'

The turning point came when Donna was twenty and in a nightclub. 'A man commented how fat I looked. It was insulting but it was also true, so I determined to lose weight, and I was slim when I met Les and we married.'

Donna continues: 'Then, while I was pregnant I got into bad habits. At main meals I used to dish up the same portions for myself as for Les (and he's tall as well as male). Now, having the children, we stay in more and Les will rent a video for us to watch, but he started bringing crisps and chocolate to eat with it! And I ate.

'Then my Gran came to live with us, and she was always baking things such as scones, bakewell tart, pies and cakes. I persuaded Gran to start at Eve's slimming group with me as she needed to lose weight for her health. We both began to lose weight, but Gran insisted on carrying on with her high-cal baking, and it was very hard for me to resist.'

But resist Donna did, 'by continually thinking "I *want* to slim"'. Then Gran moved out, so wise eating became easier.

'Now, it just comes naturally to eat this slim-fit way, for all the family. I don't force-feed the children, nor do I give them any sweety snacks between meals. What's the point of giving them bad habits that will make them suffer, as I did?'

Donna, a very wise mum as well as a wise eater and thinker, is 'back to normal' and looks and feels wonderful.

## DONNA'S PERSONAL TIPS FOR YOU

**Think Slim:** 'Save the calories for what you really enjoy.' Donna adds: 'And when you have some high-calorie enjoyment, make up for it *immediately* by cutting down on your next meals.'

**Practical Tip:** 'Sit down to eat, and eat slowly.'

Donna explains: 'This concentrates your mind on your eating, and helps you to feel satisfied with smaller portions than before.'

# BEGINNING YOUR SLIMMING

## 1 HAVE YOU ...

- Read the Seven Steps?
- Completed the Fill-in activities, including:
  a) your reasons to be slim?
  b) identifying your 'Negative Wizards'?
  c) setting your first short-term target of weight loss?
- Made some Think Slim Prompt Cards?
- Done the low-fat low-cal food shopping that you need to do?
- Bought your one-a-day multivitamin and mineral tablets?
- Got a clear idea of the Think Slim Food and Drink Programme?
  Remembered that you need to
  – weigh your portions of main foods (not low-cal veg)?
  – drink enough low-cal fluids (3 pints/9 mugs every day)?
- Decided to start some exercise? (Not absolutely essential this week, but you need to take this step soon – then plan how to do it.)
- Decided that you will make the effort to change how you think, so that you Think Slim?
- Accepted that you are *not* going on a diet?
- Accepted that you're starting on a new, better, more enjoyable 'Lifestyle for a Lifetime'?

When you have done all those things, you are ready to begin your slimming and have made the best start to help yourself to success.

## 2 WEIGH YOURSELF

You've had a lot of practice at doing that? I know from experience that dedicated dieters have a love-hate relationship with the scales as well as all sorts of (mostly unhelpful) scale strategies.

The aim of weighing yourself is to get some factual feedback about your weight-loss progress. It is not the aim to get better results so as to kid yourself that you're slimmer than you really are; nor is it to allow the scales to become the decider of your mood for the day, that is:

good weight loss = euphoria
no loss = tragedy
weight gain = catastrophe

So, please check out these 'weighing yourself' notes:

## HOW TO WEIGH
- Use good quality scales.
- Always use the same scales.
- Leave the scales in exactly the same place, or they may weigh inaccurately. (Avoid 'scale-shifting': that is, moving them around to find a floor-spot on which you weigh least!) For accuracy, the scales need to be on an even, firm surface, not a thick carpet on which you can wobble them into all sorts of weights.
- Weigh at the same time of the day, preferably first thing in the morning.
- Wear a similar weight of clothes; preferably the same clothes, or none.
- Place your feet evenly and fully on the scales (no feet overhang), and stand still. (No leaning backwards or forwards to influence the result.)
- Only weigh yourself once each week (not three times a day, before and after your bath or your binge; not again after you've exercised), because losing weight is a slow process and you will easily discourage yourself if you decide to keep hopping on and off the scales, hoping to see that needle shooting rapidly downwards – for it won't.

  Weighing too often can also prompt an unhealthy obsession with your progress. Organising your slimming needs to be a priority in your life, but your 'weight state' needs to be of no more importance than all the interesting work/hobbies/people you are involving yourself in. If your slimming, what you eat, and your weight are your only interests, they may soon become a counter-productive obsession. Make your life interesting. (Remember? 'This Is Not A Dress Rehearsal'.)
- Record your weight-loss progress on the record sheet and chart provided on pages 259–61.
- Any loss is a good loss; you are on the right track. If you lose 2 pounds/1 kilo in one week you have done extremely well; if you have lost 1 pound/½ kilo you have done very well indeed; if you have lost ½ pound/¼ kilo you have still done well.

  A loss of ½ pound/¼ kilo per week adds up towards 2 stones/13 kilos in twelve months, and that's a lot of legs, tum and bum less.

  So: Think Slim on the scales: 'Any Loss is a Good Loss.' You could print it on a card by your scales.

  Another Think Slim for the scales: 'I'm on the right track.' Repeat it to yourself at least 10 times as you leave the scales.
- Remember that, occasionally, the scales may seem not to reflect the effort you have put into your slimming.

  Scales *cannot* record your effort – only you can do that. Scales can only record your weight, and that may vary according to a number of capricious factors such as the amount of food still in your digestive tract, water retention, constipation, and a general waywardness of the body's own system. It is no use screaming that if you haven't lost weight you are giving up, and galloping off to gobble some gooey gateaux. Accept that the scales cannot always reflect your effort.

However, don't kid yourself that the scales should be showing a weight loss when it is you who didn't weigh the food portions, or you who forgot how many peanuts you'd absent-mindedly eaten.

## WOMEN: AN IMPORTANT NOTE

If you are using the 'cap' or diaphragm for contraception, a new smaller size may be needed every time you lose about 7 pounds/3 kilos in weight, or pregnancy may result. Consider using another or an additional form of contraception and consult your Birth Control adviser regularly.

## 3 AT THE END OF THE FIRST WEEK

- Weigh yourself and record the result.
- Think about your result. Congratulate yourself for any weight loss. If you have not lost weight, ask yourself why? and resolve your saboteurs for next week.
- Do a quick check through the following checklist of Think Slim good practice.

## CHECKLIST
DO YOU:
1 Drink only the Low-Cal types of soft drinks?
2 Refuse sugar in hot drinks?
3 Use low-fat spread instead of butter or margarine?
4 Have low-fat spread *or* jam/marmalade (not both)? (Or dry toast?)
5 Take a multivitamin and mineral tablet every day?
6 Eat from a smaller plate?
7 Stick to a 'No Sugar During the Day' rule?
8 Sometimes drink water/mineral water instead of other drinks?
9 Have a drink 10 minutes before you start to eat your meal?
10 Fill in your weight-loss Progress Chart?
11 Think-Slim to yourself that it's *not* slimming that's miserable, it's being fat!
12 Check food labels for sugar and saturated-fat content, and also for calorie count − *before* you buy or eat?
13 Eat *smaller* portions than you used to, except low-cal vegetables?
14 Weigh your portions of main foods, including:

bread ................ rice ................ pasta ................

potatoes ................ cereals ................ meat ................

fruit ................

(except low-cal vegetables). Tick above.
15 Make and regularly use your Think Slim Prompt Cards?

## 4  AT THE END OF EACH WEEK

- Re-weigh yourself (remembering the guidelines at the beginning of this chapter).
- Record your weight.
- Take at least a few minutes (and preferably longer) to do a Think Slim 'Review':

Did you get what you wanted from
your slimming this week?

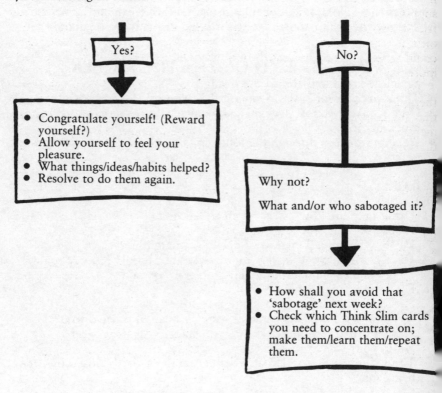

Yes?

- Congratulate yourself! (Reward yourself?)
- Allow yourself to feel your pleasure.
- What things/ideas/habits helped?
- Resolve to do them again.

No?

Why not?

What and/or who sabotaged it?

- How shall you avoid that 'sabotage' next week?
- Check which Think Slim cards you need to concentrate on; make them/learn them/repeat them.

- Re-read this Think Slim book often; choosing the section(s) that are most appropriate at the time.

## 5  TOWARDS THE END OF THE MONTH

Check the date at which you will have been slimming for one month, and write it down here:

At that time, you need to refer to Part Three; so you could also write a note for yourself on that date in your personal organiser, diary, calendar or other chosen organising system. (If you are not organised, get organised, or you cannot expect to get anything you want in life. Don't play the 'Cinders Syndrome' or 'Poor me'!)

# A SUPPORTING STEP

'I know I should be able to do it on my own,' whispers many a slimmer apologetically when they join my group.

No need to apologise. It's nonsense that we 'should' be able 'to do it on our own'. It's the words of another Negative Wizard whispering in our ear, decreeing yet another 'should' into our overloaded lives. It's Negathink instead of Slim Think.

Learning how to become slim and fit is a difficult process, and just as if we wanted to learn how to drive a car, we need both instruction and support. Maybe you have the support of someone in your family or a friend, and if that's enough for you – fine. But maybe you would like outside support. (If you live in Lincolnshire or Nottinghamshire, you could write to me for information about where I run groups, or ask for individual consultation.)

You could take this book along to a private qualified counsellor or therapist and ask that you be supported to carry out its principles. Check that the counsellor is qualified. She or he, if in Britain, could well be a member of the British Association for Counselling, and you can write to that organisation for details (refer to Useful Addresses list on page 273).

Or, if you would like the support of others who are becoming self-empowered Think-slimmers, you could organise a self-help group. For further information on this, see page 257.

## ORGANISING A SELF-HELP GROUP

- Eight to ten people is probably a reasonable size.
- Someone needs to be leader/chairperson to ensure that the group stays on the right track and doesn't become a gossip and gateau night.
- Meet once per week.
- It is best if you all agree to attend for a fixed number of weeks; at least two months for results to be worthwhile.
- It may be better not to admit anyone new for those weeks. At the end of the agreed period, you can consider who wants to continue, and admit new people.
- You could either weigh yourselves at the group, or agree on a day to weigh yourselves conveniently at home (and promise each other that you will not cheat).
- Avoid any element of competition within the group, for best weight losses etc. The idea is support, not competition.
- Support, however, does not mean sympathy mopped up with meringue gateau. You need to be honest, gentle, and tough with each other. Ask, before the group starts, if people are willing to have their eating and thinking habits criticised. That does not mean that they, as people, should be 'damned'; only their *habits* need be criticised. This is not an easy process, and if you can find someone who has had some training in group work it would be helpful to you. However, even if not, you can make efforts to follow this kind/tough approach.

- At your first meeting, spend time agreeing and writing down your group Ground Rules. These are best written big and kept on display each week. They need to look something like this:

---

1 Start time:
2 Finish time:
3 Punctuality: we agree to be punctual about starting and finishing. This is to show respect for the time of all members of the group. Our time is equally precious to each of us; we are equally important; no one has the right to waste others' time.
4 No missed meetings (unless emergency). We agree to meet for . . . weeks.
5 Talking to each other:
  – Listen to each other.
  – Confidentiality – what is said here stays here. No outside gossiping.
  – No 'put-downs'.
6 No interruptions (unless urgent).
7 No excuses.
8 Think Slim ideas will be the basis of all the meetings.
9 Every member will have a copy of the book and bring it with them each week.

---

The meetings could proceed with:
- Weighing-in. Refer to notes on weighing in this section, page 243–5. Use good quality scales.
- Feedback from each person on the weight lost.
- Feedback from each person on their progress that week in using Think Slim eating habits and thinking habits.
- Sharing of problems, and ideas to resolve them (not sympathy about how impossible it all is).
- Reading of different sections of the book, and comparing/discussing your 'fill-in' answers.

# AFTER ONE MONTH'S SLIMMING

### 1 HOW WAS IT FOR YOU?

You have reached the One Month Milestone of your slimming? Congratulations.

Research indicates that about 50 per cent of people who start slimming have given up before the end of the first month. Not you? Great. Congratulate yourself.

Or, perhaps, did you give up before that first month was up? If so, don't despair or berate yourself. Vow to start again. A baby, trying to learn how to walk, falls down many times; if she/he gave up at the first few hundred falls, she/he would be condemned to crawl through life. You had that persistence when you were a baby; you have it now. Just start again. Re-read this book, do all the fill-in exercises, and get more practice at Thinking Slim.

Settle down for a while to do a thorough Think Slim Review:
- How much weight have you lost this month?
  Enter the month's loss on your record sheet.
  Was that weight loss about what you expected?

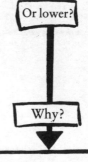

* Congratulate yourself! (Reward yourself?)
* Allow yourself to feel your pleasure.
* What things/ideas/habits helped?
* Resolve to do them again.

* Were your expectations unrealistically high?
* Were your slimming efforts sabotaged?
* What and/or who sabotaged it? Think about the saboteurs in this book (including yourself)! Make your list overleaf:

Saboteurs:

...........................................................................................................

...........................................................................................................

...........................................................................................................

★ How shall you avoid these 'saboteurs' next month? (Check ideas in this book.)

...........................................................................................................

...........................................................................................................


# 2  WHAT NEXT?
Do you want to be slimmer?                          YES?                No?

★ Absolutely sure you are not aiming too low to be healthy?
  Yes?  No?
★ Review your written 'Reasons to be Slim'. Re-motivate
  Yourself.
★ Check which Think Slim Cards you need to concentrate on;
          make them/learn them/repeat them.

  Tick when done:  _____     _____     _____

★ Decide on your next short-term weight loss target (next stone?
  7 kilos? 10 pounds? 5 kilos? and write it down: _____
★ You now have less weight to lose. Do you need to adjust your
  'Little of What You Fancy' extra indulgences allowance?
  (Between 2 stones/13 kilos and 1 stone/6 kilos: 200 calories,
  under 1 stone/6 kilos, 100 calories for two days at the
  weekends only).
★ Check at what date you will need to do your next Monthly
  review, and record it in your organising system, and here _____

                          Are You Sure? (Kidding yourself?)

                          YES      NO

                    OK:
                    Bye for now.
                    You can change your mind anytime.

# — KEEPING IT GOING —

## 1 PERSISTENCE PAYS

Stickability, that's the basis for slimming success. When you started this Think Slim programme, you were beginning on a new 'lifestyle for a lifetime', and you need to constantly remind yourself of that.

Sometimes, it will be tougher than others. That's only to be expected. Think Slim means think realistic, so it should be no surprise to you if sometimes it seems harder than other times to practise your Think Slim eating and drinking guidelines and to remember your Think Slim Prompts.

Whenever we are learning a new skill (and Think Slim is a new skill) there is a period when it is still unfamiliar, and takes effort to get it right. You may well be in that period. However, if you persist, you will move forward to the stage where the skill becomes almost second nature, and you are using it all the time without having to make any great efforts. That's when your 'Lifestyle for a Lifetime' approach really pays off.

This process is displayed in the diagram below.

LEARNING A NEW SKILL: The Think Slim Path

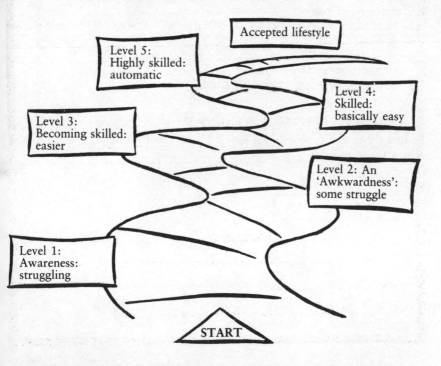

Accepted lifestyle

Level 5:
Highly skilled:
automatic

Level 4:
Skilled:
basically easy

Level 3:
Becoming skilled:
easier

Level 2: An
'Awkwardness':
some struggle

Level 1:
Awareness:
struggling

START

Remind yourself that 'if there's a set-back, you can bounce back'; and don't allow an occasional slip-up to turn into a landslide. If you find yourself slipping back into old bad eating habits or old bad negative thinking habits, take some time to yourself, with this book and some paper and a pen, and Think and write down your answers to these questions:

- What bad eating habits have I slipped into?
- What triggers them off?
- What bad thinking habits have I slipped into? (for example, 'That li'l bit won't hurt' or expecting yourself to 'be perfick'?)
- Check back over the 'Negative Wizards' section of this book to decide whether you have been allowing yourself to become a victim of any of those slimming saboteurs.

## COUNTERACT BAD HABITS WITH THINK SLIM

- Remake some suitable Think Slim Prompt Cards, and use them.
- Think of and write down plans to counteract any bad habits you have slipped into.
- Re-motivate yourself:
  - re-read your 'reasons to be slim'. Can you think of any more reasons to add to your list?
  - read a 'slimming' type magazine; look at the success stories as role models and think positive; 'if she/he can do it so can I.'
  - talk to a helpful friend/family member who will be positive and encourage you.
  - re-read the section(s) of this book that you think will be most useful to you.
  - set a new short-term weight-loss target (realistic).
  - promise yourself a reward.
  - get some exercise. Shake off the blues.

# 2 LOSING THOSE LAST FEW POUNDS OR KILOS

Losing those last persistent lumps of fat can be hard work. First, do you still want to lose it?

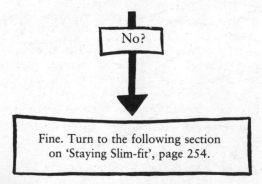

No?

Fine. Turn to the following section on 'Staying Slim-fit', page 254.

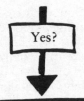

Now ask yourself critically whether you have set your total weight-loss target realistically. You are not aiming too low, are you? Check these points:
- Is your aim to be slim, or to be thin-thin-model-thin? (If you are still aiming for thin go back and re-read Negative Wizards in our Culture 'Never too thin' (see page 58), and then do yourself a favour and reset your target more realistically, more freely and more wisely. (Remember 'bound feet'? You don't remember? Then read that Negative Wizard again, and again, and again, until you have freed yourself, or go and seek some counselling, now.)
- Is your best friend telling you that you are slim enough? (As long as you are sure she/he is a best friend . . .)

If you are sure that your target is wise and realistic, you need to concentrate your thinking and your action towards plans for losing that last amount of excess weight:
- Review your eating habits:
  - can you cut out any more 'fatty' food?
  - are you weighing your portions? and eating the right quantities according to the Food and Drink Programme?
  - are you still including alcohol? You could choose to say 'No' until you have reached your target.
  - you probably need to exclude your extra 'little fancy' foods for a while.
  - You would succeed more easily if you chose to increase your exercise level. Don't massively increase it suddenly, but you could exercise every day, and adjust the time depending on what you do now. For example: make it 30 minutes aerobic activity (cycling, swimming, very brisk walking) instead of 20 minutes; or 45 minutes instead of 30, or one hour instead of 45 minutes.
  - focus on your Think Slim Prompt Cards (make some new ones?) to increase your motivation and keep your thoughts on the right

(positive) track.
- take one day at a time – don't distress yourself wondering how long it will take.
- plan yourself a treat (preferably non-food/drink) as a reward for all your extra efforts.
- Keep at it; 'stickability' will win you through.

## RED LETTER DAY

Hurrah! Hurrah! Hurrah! This is the day that you have worked towards, the target you set yourself to achieve, and you have achieved it. It is a superb achievement, so you are entitled to feel proud of yourself as well as delighted.

Mark your record sheet with a big red-letter 'T' for Target. If you wish, mark your diary too, your calendar, your dog's collar, your spouse's shirt sleeve . . . anything . . . anywhere . . . Let the playful child inside of you out to play . . . Hug someone, dance, laugh, cry.

Reward yourself as you had planned.

I'm delighted for you. Life's too Short to Live it Fat. Now you've joined the ranks of the Slim-fitters who can really enjoy and make the most of their lives.

# 3  A LIFESTYLE FOR A LIFETIME: STAYING SLIM-FIT, ENJOYING LIFE

Congratulations on reaching the Target of weight loss that you set yourself; it's a magnificent achievement. Now you can enjoy your success.

The 7 Steps of this Think Slim programme have emphasised that you have been starting on a lifestyle for a lifetime, and that is what you can continue to do now.

You have not been on a diet, and so you have no need to think about going 'off' a diet and back to your 'normal' eating habits. Those old 'normal' eating habits were in fact your 'overweight' eating habits and if you choose to go back to them, you will be choosing to go back to being overweight.

However, you have learned to Think Slim, and to find new normal eating and exercising habits; and the way to enjoy slim-fit living is to continue with your new lifestyle for a lifetime.

So, carry on:
- The same ways of thinking
- The same low-fat, low-calorie, low-sugar, high-fibre shopping
- The same low-fat cooking principles
- The same exercise guidelines
  But change:
- Increase your food in moderation; an excellent system is to continue in the same relatively stringent way during the week and increase

your food treats at the weekend (two days only) by only 250 or so calories each day. You need to experiment to find out what's possible for you without gaining excessive amounts of weight.

- Check your weight once each week.
- Think of aiming to stay within a range of about 2 pounds/1 kilo under and 4 pounds/2 kilos over your target weight now achieved, for it is unrealistic to expect your weight to remain exactly the same all the time.
- As soon as your weight reaches those few pounds/kilos over your target, apply your Think Slim principles strictly to overcome the excess weight.
- Allow yourself to feel confident about reducing any weight gain which may be due to holidays or celebrations. Refer again to the appropriate sections of this book to help you.
- After a little while, all the compliments and congratulations from others will stop and you will have only yourself to sustain your interest in staying slim. Yourself is enough. The self-empowered slimmer does not depend on others for her/his motivation. Constantly re-motivate yourself, reminding yourself of the Think Slim philosophy that 'Life's Too Short to Live it Fat', that 'Life in the Fat Lane is life in the Lack-lustre Lane', and that you'll 'Never go Back to the Fat Old Ways and the Fat Old Days'.
- I wish you joy. I wish that you enjoy yourself in your self-empowered and responsible way, making the most of your slim-fit life. You deserve it and are entitled to accept it.

This is Not A Dress Rehearsal; it's now or never. I don't wish you luck, because encouraging you to wait for luck would be encouraging you to wait, like Cinders, for life. Make your own life, and keep it balanced with work, rest, play, and positive relationships. Treat yourself with respect as you do others, and demand that they treat you with respect – refuse to accept the unacceptable.

Neither ponder morosely over the past, nor wishful-think for the future. Think slim and Think carefully what else you want and where you want to be, then plan and act to reach those things. Don't try to Do-It-All, but do what is most dear to you – and *you* choose.

# —— A THINK SLIM —— OFFER

'I wish I could take you home with me!' many a new slimmer has lamented to me.

Well, now you can. You can order an audio-cassette which will help to support you in your Think Slim slim-fitness campaign.

Side 1 can be played any time at your convenience (including in the car), and reminds you of the fundamental ideas of this approach, and the Think Slim prompts.

Side 2 is designed for you to play as a relaxation exercise. This will enable you to learn and remember the approaches to relaxation even more effectively. Also, it will help you to cope better – rested, relaxed and with renewed energy – with the stresses of everyday life. This side of the tape should *not* be used while you are driving a vehicle, or while you are in the bath.

The tape has clear instructions. All you need to do is relax and listen; you will learn quicker, and feel better than you could have imagined.

To order a copy of the *Think Slim Relax and Learn* audio cassette tape, simply send your name and address with a cheque for £8.99 (£6.99 plus £2 postage and packing – Britain only) to:

Eve Brock, Think Slim, PO Box 22, Gainsborough, Lincs DN21 5PP.

## THINK SLIM – BY POST
You can follow a Think Slim Programme, based on this book but with the added support of personal advice for your own lifestyle, by joining the Think Slim Postal Programme.

You will complete a questionnaire to explain your individual circumstances, receive advice tailored to you personally, and be able to contact your expert adviser by phone each week. For full details (Britain only), please write to:

Eve Brock, Think Slim Postal Programme.

## WHEN YOU'VE LOST WEIGHT THE THINK SLIM WAY
You could help others, and run your own group. Send to the address above for details.

# RECORD SHEETS AND CHARTS

## WEIGHT-LOSS RECORD SHEET

| Date | Weight | Weight Lost This Week | Weight Lost This Month | Comments |
|------|--------|----------------------|------------------------|----------|
|      |        |                      |                        |          |
|      |        |                      |                        |          |
|      |        |                      |                        |          |
|      |        |                      |                        |          |
|      |        |                      |                        |          |
|      |        |                      |                        |          |
|      |        |                      |                        |          |
|      |        |                      |                        |          |
|      |        |                      |                        |          |
|      |        |                      |                        |          |
|      |        |                      |                        |          |
|      |        |                      |                        |          |
|      |        |                      |                        |          |
|      |        |                      |                        |          |
|      |        |                      |                        |          |
|      |        |                      |                        |          |
|      |        |                      |                        |          |
|      |        |                      |                        |          |
|      |        |                      |                        |          |

| Enter your weight (in stones) in this space | lb | | | | | |
|---|---|---|---|---|---|---|
| | 12 | | | | | |
| | 10 | | | | | |
| | 8 | | | | | |
| | 6 | | | | | |
| | 4 | | | | | |
| | 2 | | | | | |
| Enter your weight (in stones) in this space | lb | | | | | |
| | 12 | | | | | |
| | 10 | | | | | |
| | 8 | | | | | |
| | 6 | | | | | |
| | 4 | | | | | |
| | 2 | | | | | |
| Enter your weight (in stones) in this space | lb | | | | | |
| | 12 | | | | | |
| | 10 | | | | | |
| | 8 | | | | | |
| | 6 | | | | | |
| | 4 | | | | | |
| | 2 | | | | | |
| WEEK | | 1 | 2 | 3 | 4 | |

| | | | | | | 7 | 8 | 9 | 10 | 11 | 12 |
|---|---|---|---|---|---|---|---|---|---|---|---|

**SLIMFIT Weight-Loss Progress Chart**

# MEASUREMENT RECORD

| Date | Chest/Bust | Waist | Hips | Thighs |
|------|-----------|-------|------|--------|
|      |           |       |      |        |
|      |           |       |      |        |
|      |           |       |      |        |
|      |           |       |      |        |
|      |           |       |      |        |
|      |           |       |      |        |
|      |           |       |      |        |
|      |           |       |      |        |
|      |           |       |      |        |
| TOTAL LOSS |      |       |      |        |

Between _____

And _____

# SLIM-FIT FOOD AND DRINK DIARY

Date: _____

**Important:** Weigh/measure your portions. (*Guesses mean extra food – and extra-fat YOU!*)

Calories need only be entered for your 'Little bit of what you fancy' extras, but, if you wish, count them all.

| | Morning food & drink | cal | Afternoon food & drink | cal | Evening/night food & drink | cal |
|---|---|---|---|---|---|---|
| M O N | | | | | | |
| T U E | | | | | | |
| W E D | | | | | | |
| T H U | | | | | | |
| F R I | | | | | | |
| S A T | | | | | | |
| S U N | | | | | | |

How was it for you? Think about your week; consider any good ideas/ habits, *and* also any that are unhelpful.

Your Comments: ........................................................................................

# —— QUIZ ANSWERS ——

## CHRISTMAS CALORIE QUIZ: ANSWERS

|  | *Approx Calories* |
|---|---|
| 1 oz/28 g stuffed olives | 45 |
| 1 peanut | 5 |
| 1 oz/28 g peanuts, roasted and salted | 168 |
| 1 oz/28 g roast turkey (no skin) | 40 |
| 1 oz/28 g roast duck (no skin) | 54 |
| 1 large roast potato | 200 |
| 5 oz/150 g Christmas pudding | 425 |
| 1 oz/28 g brandy butter | 150 |
| 3½ oz/100 g Christmas cake | 350 |
| 1 mince pie | 200–250 |
| 1 luxury chocolate | 50 |
| 1 oz/28 g shortbread | 140 |
| 1 grape | 5 |
| 1 oz/28 g grapes (black or green) | 18 |
| 1 tangerine (c. 3½ oz/100 g) | 35 |
| 1 oz/28 g fresh dates | 40 |
| 1 oz/28 gdates, dried with stones | 60 |
| 1 oz/28 g Brazil nuts (shelled) | 175 |
| 1 oz/28 g walnuts (shelled) | 147 |
| 1 oz/28 g chestnuts (shelled) | 48 |

## BASIC CALORIE-COUNT QUIZ: ANSWERS

|  | *Approx Calories* |
|---|---|
| 1 oz/28 g butter | 210 |
| 1 oz/28 g margarine | 210 |
| 1 oz/28 g full fat hard cheese | 120 |
| 1 oz/28 g shortcrust pastry, when cooked | 150 |
| 1 oz/28 g wholemeal bread | 65 |
| 2 oz/56 g potato, when cooked | 45 |
| 2 oz/56 g brown rice, when cooked | 65 |
| 2 oz/56 g wholewheat pasta, when cooked | 85 |
| 1 medium egg, white only | 10 |
| 1 medium egg, yolk only | 70 |

1 oz/28 g lean beef, when cooked                                    47
1 oz/28 g lean chicken, without skin, when cooked                   40
1 oz/28 g chicken, including skin, when cooked                      60

1 oz/28 g milk chocolate                                           150

# PROMPTS QUIZ ANSWERS

## YOUR ESCHATOLOGICAL THINK SLIM LIST
From quiz on page 229.
FUNDAMENTAL THINK SLIM
1 The key to being slim is: THINK SLIM.
2 I THINK therefore I am . . . slim-fit.
3 Life – this is not a DRESS REHEARSAL. Live now, there is no 'later'.
4 Life in the Fat Lane is life in SLOW MOTION.
5 Slim-fit living is more ENJOYABLE living.
6 Life *isn't* FAIR.
7 Nobody promised me that life would be FAIR.
8 Choosing to do one thing often means choosing NOT to do another.
9 *Everything* in life is EASIER said than done.

ON EATING
1 'A LITTLE of What You Fancy Does You Good!' (A LITTLE only: a LOT makes you Fat!)
2 Think before you eat a THING.
3 If the FOOD'S not fabulous don't WASTE the calories on it!
4 Those who OVER-INDULGE – *bulge!*
5 You'll get more PLEASURE out of being slim than you ever got from OVER-EATING.
6 It's just as FATTENING If You Eat it In SECRET.
7 Linger LONGER with your food. Get more PLEASURE out of LESS calories.
8 Food can't solve PROBLEMS. Only I can do that.
9 More FOOD can only make me more fat.
10 I give up to GET.

ON SLIMMING
1 We are overweight because we OVER-EAT.
2 Make EFFORTS – not EXCUSES.
3 It's not SLIMMING that's miserable – it's being FAT!
4 Deprived. Who's MOST Deprived? (The slim person who deprives herself only of over-eating – *or* the fat one who eats anything and everything and deprives herself of the pleasures of being slim?)
5 Successful slimmers MAKE it happen; disastrous dieters LET it happen.

ON FAILURE

1 You won't know where you're going, if you're always LOOKING back.
2 You haven't failed until you STOP TRYING.

ON EATING OUT

1 I've paid for it, I've got to eat it: No! I've paid for it so I can DO WHAT I LIKE with it – and that includes LEAVING it!

# HOW MUCH HAVE YOU LEARNED SO FAR?
## ANSWERS
From quiz on page 230.

1 We are overweight because we OVER-EAT.
2 We should keep on weighing our FOOD, NOT OURSELVES.
3 It's good to make resolutions and set targets, but these should be REALISTIC.
4 Lil is plagued by a Negative Wizard herself; she used to think: 'That li'l bit won't HURT!'
    Was she right?
    *No.* Every calorie we eat is counted by our body, if not by us. What we eat, we work off, or wear!
5 An extra 50 Calories a day could amount to over 4 stones/25 kilos of weight gain in 10 years.
6 One peanut contains 5 calories.
    One grape contains 5 calories (or maybe 10, if it's an extra large species.)
    Butter, margarine, and polyunsaturated spread (such as Flora) all have the same amount of calories: 210 in 1 oz/28 g.
7 Motivators: Think WHY and Think POSSIBLE.
    Think Why is thinking about your reasons for slimming; working out the advantages of being slim.
    Think Possible is thinking that it is POSSIBLE for you to become slim, no matter whether you have failed before.
8 Two words/phrases, beginning with P, which are MOST important for slimmers are PERSISTENCE and POSITIVE ATTITUDE.
9 It is a good idea for slimmers to take a vitamin and mineral tablet each day because it is not easy for a slimmer, on a restricted daily intake of calories (for a woman, between 1000–1400 calories) to be certain of getting all she/he needs. This is particularly so because of personal food preferences. (Not many of us regularly choose spinach!) It is also because considerable amounts of vitamins are lost in preparation, cooking, and due to produce not being as fresh as is ideal.
    Are you taking yours?! If your answer is no, ask yourself why not?

You need to be sure that you are fit as well as becoming slimmer, so you need to take it daily. If forgetfulness is your problem, decide on a time each day when you will take the tablet. Write yourself a large note and stick it up somewhere you will be certain to see it, near where your tablets are kept. Soon you will remember automatically. Or, you could put the week's supply out somewhere convenient and obvious – but *not* within the reach of children.

10  DO'S AND DON'TS!
Don't BORE yourself with cottage cheese and carrots all week!
Don't make yourself MISERABLE over a small weight loss.
Do think that you are 'on the RIGHT TRACK!'
Any (sensible) weight loss is a GOOD loss.
Do drink enough liquids (low-calorie). How many mugs each day? NINE.
Do make your eating HIGH-FIBRE.
   Why? Because it has filling-power, and is healthy for your digestive and bowel system.
And by eating which foods? High-fibre cereals, wholemeal bread, wholemeal pasta, brown rice; vegetables, including potatoes in their jackets; pulses; fruit.

11  Have you felt hungry this week?

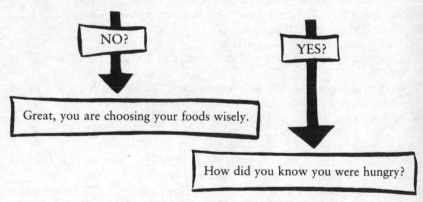

NO?

Great, you are choosing your foods wisely.

YES?

How did you know you were hungry?

I hope that you didn't answer that you knew because you could have murdered for a Big Mac. Such food longings are probably just lust, and we all experience it from time to time! If you are hungry you would have a real physical stomach sensation, often accompanied by a tell-tale rumble.
   What did you do about it? I hope that, first, you had a low-calorie drink. Then you stopped to think, Think Slim: 'Am I really hungry, or is it just lust?'
   If it was hunger – did you think some more, about what you should eat, and choose wisely? Complex carbohydrates, (such as wholemeal

crispbread, bread, pasta, rice, and potato), plus vegetables, possess good filling power at a relatively cheap cost in calories, whereas fats (butter, margarines, cakes, biscuits, pastry, red meats and rich sauces) are especially talented at fattening.

In a hurry, need fast food? Fruit is the fastest, wisest food for the hurrying hungry slimmer.

**After Checking Your Knowledge:** if you found that in any of the areas highlighted by this quiz your knowledge is weak, skim back through the book and re-read those areas. Having knowledge is the first stage for successful slimming.

# THINK SLIM SLIMMING

This is to certify that

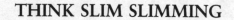

achieved her PERSONAL TARGET

on . . . . . . .

having lost . . . . . in weight,

as promised

She is a Person Who
Sets A Target
Works for It
and
Gets It!

*CONGRATULATIONS!*
*A GREAT ACHIEVEMENT!*

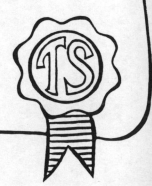

# THINK SLIM PROMPTS

Photocopy this page to make your own 'instant' Think Slim Prompt Cards.

DO I REALLY WANT IT?
NO I DON'T.
SHALL I EAT IT?
NO I WON'T!

IF I HAVE A SETBACK,
I BOUNCE BACK

I USED TO BE A
DIETING DISASTER.
NOW I'M A
SUCCESSFUL SLIMMER

I AM A PERSON
WHO SETS A TARGET,
WORKS AT IT
AND
GETS IT

THIS IS NOT A DRESS
REHEARSAL.
LIFE'S TOO SHORT TO
LIVE IT FAT.
MAKE EFFORTS, NOT
EXCUSES!

FOOD CAN'T SOLVE
PROBLEMS.
ONLY I CAN DO THAT

SUCCESSFUL
SLIMMERS MAKE IT
HAPPEN!
I CAN MAKE IT
HAPPEN!

IT'S NOT SLIMMING
THAT'S MISERABLE –
IT'S BEING FAT!

# — USEFUL ADDRESSES — IN BRITAIN

## ALCOHOL-RELATED PROBLEMS
Alcoholics Anonymous
11 Redcliffe Gardens, London SW10 9GB. Tel: 071 352 3001

Al-Anon Family Groups
61 Great Dover St, London SE1 4YF. Tel: 071 403 0888

## COUNSELLING SUPPORT
British Association for Counselling
37a Sheep St, Rugby, Warwicks. Tel: 0788 578328

## EATING DISORDERS
Anorexic Aid (also for Bulimia sufferers)
The Priory Centre, 11 Priory Rd, High Wycombe, Bucks.
Tel: 0494 521431

Anorexic Family Aid (also for Bulimia Sufferers)
Sackville Place, 44 Magdalen St, Norwich, Norfolk NJ3 1JE.

The Maisner Centre for Eating Disorders
PO Box 464, Hove, East Sussex BN3 2BN.

## MENOPAUSE & HRT INFORMATION
Amarant Trust
80 Lambeth Rd, London SE1 7PW. Tel: 071 401 3855

HRT Information Line, 24 hours Tel: 0836 400 190

Women's Health Concern Ltd
PO Box 1629, London W8 6AU. Tel: 071 938 3932

## RELATIONSHIPS
Relate (Previously known as Marriage Guidance Council. Provides
counselling.) Local branch should be in your phone book, or contact:
Herbert Gray College, Little Church St, Rugby, Warwicks CV21 3AP.
Tel: 0788 573241

Both of the following organisations will supply you with their approved list of
private counsellors who can help with relationship issues:
British Association for Counselling
37a Sheep St, Rugby, Warwicks EV1 38X. Tel: 0788 578328

Association of Sexual and Marital Therapists (ASMT)
PO Box 62, Sheffield S10 3TS.

SEXUAL ABUSE
Kate Adams Crisis Centre. Offers help to adults who have been abused as children; and to parents of abused children. Tel: 081 593 9428

Rape Crisis Centre
See local phone book, or phone head office on 071 837 1600.

Women's Therapy Centre
6 Manor Gardens, London N7. Tel: 071 263 6200

STRESS MANAGEMENT
Relaxation for Living (Classes nationwide and correspondence courses.)
29 Burnwood Park Rd, Walton on Thames, Surrey KT12 5LH.

The Society of the Teachers of The Alexander Technique (Also for posture and problems with the spine/back.)
20 London House, 266 Fulham Rd, London SW10 9EL. Tel: 071 351 0828

STUDY COURSES
Healthy Eating. At-home study course (not degree level).
The Open University, PO Box 188, Milton Keynes MK7 6AA.

'Look After Yourself'. A general healthy eating, fitness and coronary attack prevention Programme.
The Health Education Authority. Local branch may be in the phone book or contact: 78 New Oxford St, London WC1A 1AH. Tel: 071 637 1881

VIOLENCE
The Women's Aid Federation (WAFE)
PO Box 391, Bristol, Avon BS99 7WS. Tel: 0272 633 542
OR London Branch, Fetherstone St, London EC1Y 8RT. Tel: 071 251 6537

Men's Centre. Offers re-education programmes for men who are violent to women. Tel: 071 267 8713

WOMEN'S ASSISTANCE (Eating Disorders, and other issues)
Women's Therapy Centre
6 Manor Gardens, London N7. Tel: 071 263 6200

WOMEN'S HEALTH
National Association for Pre-Menstrual Syndrome
23 Upper Park Rd, Kingston Upon Thames, Surrey KT2 5LB.

Pre-Menstrual Tension Advisory Service
PO Box 268, Hove, East Sussex BN3 1RW. Tel: 0273 771366

Well Woman Clinic (No doctor's referral necessary.)
Marie Stopes House, 108 Whitfield St, London W1. Tel: 071 388 0662

# —— MORE SUPPORT ——
# FURTHER READING

ASSERTIVENESS
*A Woman in Your Own Right* Anne Dickson (Quartet, 1982)

COOKERY BOOKS
*Low-Fat and No-Fat Cooking* Jackie Applebee (Thorsons, 1989)
*Light and Easy: Over 350 Quick and Healthy Low Calorie Recipes* Barbara
Gibbons (Harper Collins, 1992)
*Slimming Menus* Audrey Ellis (Sampson Low, 1979)
*Slim Cuisine Diet: Twenty-eight Days That Will Change Your Life* Sue
Kreitzman (Ebury Press, 1991)
*The Low-Fat Special Diet Cookbook: 100 Delicious Ways to Cut Right Down
on Fat* Sarah Bounds (Thorsons, 1991)
*365 Slim & Healthy Dishes,* Ebury All Colour Collection (Ebury Press, 1992)

COPING
*Doing It Now* Edwin C. Bliss (Futura, 1990)
(A 'stop procrastinating, get on with it, how to' book.)

DEALING WITH DEPRESSION
*Depression: The Way Out of Your Prison* Dorothy Rowe (Routledge & Kegan
Paul, 1989)

EATING DISORDERS
*Feasting and Fasting* Paulette Maisner (Fontana, 1985)
*The Art of Starvation: An Adolescence Observed* Sheila MacLeod (Virago,
1981)
*Anorexia Nervosa: Let Me Be* AH Crisp (Bailliere, 1990)
*Hunger Strike* Susie Orbach (Faber & Faber, 1986)
*Coping With Bulimia* Barbara French (Thorsons, 1987)

EXERCISE
*Aquarobics: Getting Fit and Keeping Fit in the Swimming Pool* Glenda Baum
(Arrow, 1991)

GENERAL HEALTH
*Our Bodies, Ourselves: A Health Book by and for Women* Angela Phillips
and Jill Rakusen (Penguin, 1989)
*Getting Well Again* O Carl Simonton, Stephanie Matthews-Simonton and
James L Creighton (Bantam Books, 1986)

MENOPAUSE AND HRT
*The Amarant Book of Hormone Replacement Therapy* (Available from the
Amarant Trust, 80 Lambeth Rd, London SE1 7PW. Other publications and
information available, tel: 071 401 3855.)

PERIODS AND PRE-MENSTRUAL SYNDROME
*Pre-Menstrual Syndrome* Caroline Shreeve (Thorsons, 1983)
*Lifting the Curse (Self Help for Aches, Pains, Cramps and Other Monthly
Miseries)* Beryl Kingston (Sheldon Press, 1980)
*Beat Pre-Menstrual Tension Through Diet* Maryon Stewart (Ebury Press,
1990)

RELATIONSHIPS
*The Relate Guide to Better Relationships* Sarah Litvinoff (Ebury Press, 1991)
(Don't wait for problems to occur in relationships. If you read nothing else,
read this book.)

SEXUALITY
Aimed towards women:
*The Mirror Within: a New Look at Sexuality* Anne Dickson (Quartet, 1985)
*Female Desire: Women's Sexuality Today* Rosalind Coward (Paladin, 1984)
Sexuality, General:
*Coping with Sexual Relationships* Judy Greenwood (MacDonald, 1984)
*Sexual Happiness: A Practical Approach* Yaffe, Maurice & Fenwick, Elizabeth
(Dorling Kindersley, 1986)

STRESS MANAGEMENT
*Book of Stress Survival: How to Relax and De-stress Your Life* Alix Kirsta
(Unwin, 1986)
*The Art of Changing: A New Approach to the Alexander Technique* Glen
Park (Ashgrove Press, 1988)
*The Joy of Stress* Dr P Hanson (Pan, 1988)

WOMEN'S LIVES
*The Good Girl Syndrome: How Women Are Programmed to Fail in a Man's
World – and How to Stop It* William Fezler (Thorson Grapevine, 1988)
*Women Who Love Too Much* Robin Norwood (Arrow, 1986)

# INDEX

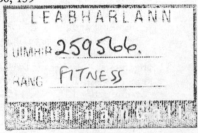